175 Popular Dairy-Free Recipes

(175 Popular Dairy-Free Recipes - Volume 1)

Caroline Riffe

Content

CHAPTER 4: DAIRY-FREE SNACK RECIPES 47

CHAPTER 5: DAIRY-FREE CAKE RECIPES 58

CHAPTER 6: DAIRY-FREE DESSERT RECIPES 70

CHAPTER 7: DAIRY-FREE KIDS' RECIPES 80

CHAPTER 8: AWESOME DAIRY-FREE RECIPES.. 93

Chapter 1: Dairy-Free Breakfast Recipes

***

1. All In One Baked Mushrooms

Serving: 2 | Prep: 5mins | Cook: 25mins |Ready in:

Ingredients

- 2 tbsp olive oil
- 4 very large field mushrooms
- 4 slices good-quality cooked ham
- 4 eggs

Direction

- Heat oven to 220C/fan 200C/gas 7. Drizzle a little olive oil over the base of a ceramic baking dish, then pop in the mushrooms.
- Drizzle with the remaining oil and seasoning. Bake for 15 mins until soft, then remove from the oven.
- Tuck the ham slices around the mushrooms to create little pockets. Crack the eggs into the pockets, then return to the oven for 10 mins until the egg white is set and the yolk is still a little runny. Serve scooped straight from the dish. Great with baked beans and chips.

Nutrition Information

- Calories: 379 calories
- Saturated Fat: 6 grams saturated fat
- Fiber: 3 grams fiber
- Sodium: 1.79 milligram of sodium
- Protein: 30 grams protein
- Total Carbohydrate: 1 grams carbohydrates
- Sugar: 1 grams sugar
- Total Fat: 28 grams fat

2. Asparagus Soldiers With A Soft Boiled Egg

Serving: 4 | Prep: 10mins | Cook: 10mins |Ready in:

Ingredients

- 1 tbsp olive oil
- 50g fine dry breadcrumbs
- pinch each chilliand paprika
- 16-20 asparagus spears
- 4 eggs

Direction

- Heat the oil in a pan, add the breadcrumbs, then fry until crisp and golden. Season with the spices and flaky sea salt, then leave to cool. Cook the asparagus in a large pan of boiling salted water for 3-5 mins until tender. At the same time, boil the eggs for 3-4 mins. Put each egg in an egg cup on a plate. Drain the asparagus and divide between plates. Scatter over the crumbs and serve.

Nutrition Information

- Calories: 186 calories
- Saturated Fat: 2 grams saturated fat
- Total Carbohydrate: 12 grams carbohydrates
- Sugar: 3 grams sugar
- Protein: 12 grams protein
- Total Fat: 10 grams fat
- Fiber: 2 grams fiber
- Sodium: 0.72 milligram of sodium

3. Baked Eggs With Ham & Spinach

Serving: 2 | Prep: 10mins | Cook: 30mins |Ready in:

Ingredients

- 1 tbsp olive oil
- 1 small onion, finely chopped
- 1 garlic clove, crushed
- 1 small green chilli, deseeded and finely chopped
- 400g can chopped tomato
- 100g ready-roasted pepper from a jar, drained and sliced
- 180g pack ham, torn, or shredded ham hock
- 50g baby spinach
- 2 medium eggs
- pinch cayenne pepper
- crusty bread, to serve

Direction

- Heat oven to 180C/160C fan/gas 4. Heat the oil in a small ovenproof sauté pan. Add the onion and cook for 6 mins until softened. Stir in the garlic and chilli, and cook for a couple mins more. Add the tomatoes and 100ml water. Season well and stir through the peppers and ham. Bring to a simmer and cook for 10 mins until the sauce has started to thicken. Add the spinach, stirring through to wilt.
- Make 2 hollows in the sauce and crack your eggs into them. Add a pinch of cayenne, transfer to the oven and bake for 10 mins until the whites of the eggs have set. Serve straight away with crusty bread.

Nutrition Information

- Calories: 300 calories
- Total Carbohydrate: 11 grams carbohydrates
- Fiber: 3 grams fiber
- Sugar: 8 grams sugar
- Protein: 29 grams protein
- Total Fat: 16 grams fat

- Saturated Fat: 4 grams saturated fat
- Sodium: 2.9 milligram of sodium

4. Baked Eggs With Spinach & Tomato

Serving: Serves 4 | Prep: 5mins | Cook: 15mins |Ready in:

Ingredients

- 100g bag spinach
- 400g can chopped tomatoes
- 1 tsp chilli flakes
- 4 eggs

Direction

- Heat oven to 200C/180C fan/gas 6. Put the spinach into a colander, then pour over a kettle of boiling water to wilt the leaves. Squeeze out excess water and divide between 4 small ovenproof dishes.
- Mix the tomatoes with the chilli flakes and some seasoning, then add to the dishes with the spinach. Make a small well in the centre of each and crack in an egg. Bake for 12-15 mins or more depending on how you like your eggs. Serve with crusty bread, if you like.

Nutrition Information

- Calories: 114 calories
- Sodium: 0.43 milligram of sodium
- Saturated Fat: 2 grams saturated fat
- Sugar: 2 grams sugar
- Protein: 9 grams protein
- Total Carbohydrate: 3 grams carbohydrates
- Fiber: 2 grams fiber
- Total Fat: 7 grams fat

5. Better Than Baked Beans With Spicy Wedges

Serving: 2 | Prep: 10mins | Cook: 35mins | Ready in:

Ingredients

- 1 tsp oil
- 1 onion, halved and thinly sliced
- 2 rashers streaky bacon, cut into large-ish pieces
- 1 tsp sugar, brown if you have it
- 400g can chopped tomato
- 200ml stock from a cube
- 410g can cannellini bean, butter or haricot beans in water
- For the wedges
- 1 tbsp white flour (plain or self-raising)
- 0.5 tsp cayenne pepper, paprika or mild chilli powder
- 1 tsp dried mixed herb (optional)
- 2 baking potatoes, each cut into 8 wedges
- 2 tsp oil

Direction

- Heat oven to 200C/fan 180C/gas 6. For the wedges, mix the flour, cayenne and herbs (if using), add some salt and pepper, then toss with the potatoes and oil until well coated. Tip into a roasting tin, then bake for about 35 mins until crisp and cooked through.
- Meanwhile, heat the oil in a non-stick pan, then gently fry the onion and bacon together for 5-10 mins until the onions are softened and just starting to turn golden. Stir in the sugar, tomatoes, stock and seasoning to taste, then simmer the sauce for 5 mins. Add the beans, then simmer for another 5 mins until the sauce has thickened. Serve with the wedges.

Nutrition Information

- Calories: 399 calories
- Protein: 19 grams protein
- Sodium: 1.14 milligram of sodium
- Total Fat: 11 grams fat
- Saturated Fat: 2 grams saturated fat
- Total Carbohydrate: 60 grams carbohydrates
- Sugar: 15 grams sugar

6. Coconut Crêpes With Raspberry Sauce

Serving: 6 | Prep: 10mins | Cook: 25mins | Ready in:

Ingredients

- For the raspberry sauce
- 200g raspberries
- 2 tsp cornflour
- 2 tsp maple syrup
- For the coconut crêpes
- 140g plain flour
- 2 large eggs
- 300ml coconut milk
- 2 tbsp toasted desiccated coconut
- a little sunflower oil, for frying

Direction

- Set aside 6 of the raspberries. Mix the cornflour with 1 tbsp water until smooth. Measure 300ml water in a pan, and stir in the cornflour paste. Heat, stirring, until thickened. Add the remaining raspberries and cook gently, mashing the berries to a pulp. Strain the mixture through a sieve into a bowl to remove the seeds, pushing through as much of the mixture as you can. Quarter the reserved raspberries and add to the sauce, along with the maple syrup.
- To make the crêpes, tip the flour and a pinch of salt into a large jug, then beat in the eggs, coconut milk, 200ml water and 11/2 tbsp toasted coconut to make a batter the consistency of double cream. Thin with a little more water if it is too thick. Heat a small frying pan with a dash of oil, then pour in a little batter, swirling the pan so that it completely covers the base. Leave to set over the heat for 1 min, then carefully flip it over

and cook the other side for a few secs more. Transfer to a plate and repeat with the remaining batter until you have at least 12. Stir the batter to redistribute the coconut as you use it. Serve 2 crêpes per person with a drizzle of the sauce and a little of the remaining toasted coconut.

Nutrition Information

- Calories: 265 calories
- Fiber: 3 grams fiber
- Sodium: 0.2 milligram of sodium
- Total Fat: 15 grams fat
- Sugar: 4 grams sugar
- Protein: 6 grams protein
- Saturated Fat: 11 grams saturated fat
- Total Carbohydrate: 24 grams carbohydrates

Pour in the egg mixture and cook, stirring occasionally over the heat. Once it's almost set flip over to cook the other side for a few seconds more.

- Halve the baps and squash on the tomatoes, quarter the omelette and serve, 2 pieces inside each bap.

Nutrition Information

- Calories: 323 calories
- Fiber: 4 grams fiber
- Sugar: 4 grams sugar
- Total Carbohydrate: 24 grams carbohydrates
- Protein: 19 grams protein
- Sodium: 1 milligram of sodium
- Total Fat: 16 grams fat
- Saturated Fat: 4 grams saturated fat

7. Egg & Tomato Baps

Serving: 2 | Prep: 5mins | Cook: 5mins | Ready in:

Ingredients

- 2 tomatoes, halved
- 2 tsp olive oil
- 4 eggs
- couple sprigs parsley, chopped
- 1 garlic clove, finely chopped
- 2 wholewheat baps

Direction

- Brush the cut side of the tomatoes with a little of the oil then cook them on a low heat, cut-side down in a small, non-stick frying pan. While they cook, beat the eggs with seasoning and the chopped parsley in a small bowl. Turn the tomatoes over to briefly heat on the other side and then set aside.
- Wipe the pan, then add the remaining oil and cook the garlic on a medium heat for a few seconds, stirring all the time until softened.

8. Grapefruit, Agave & Pistachio Salad

Serving: 2 | Prep: 5mins | Cook: | Ready in:

Ingredients

- 1 pink grapefruit
- 1 white grapefruit
- 1 tbsp agave nectar
- 1 tsp chopped pistachio

Direction

- Segment grapefruits, removing as much of the pith as possible. Divide the segments between two bowls and top with with agave and pistachios.

Nutrition Information

- Calories: 107 calories
- Total Carbohydrate: 21 grams carbohydrates
- Sugar: 12 grams sugar
- Fiber: 2 grams fiber

- Protein: 2 grams protein
- Total Fat: 1 grams fat

- Sugar: 3 grams sugar
- Protein: 34 grams protein
- Sodium: 0.56 milligram of sodium
- Total Fat: 24 grams fat

9. Minty Salmon & Broccoli Frittata

Serving: 4 | Prep: 5mins | Cook: 25mins | Ready in:

Ingredients

- 500g new potato
- 1 small head broccoli, cut into florets
- 2 skinless salmon fillets
- 1 tbsp olive oil
- small handful mint, finely chopped
- 8 eggs, beaten

Direction

- Boil potatoes in a large pan for 10-12 mins, adding the broccoli pieces for the final 4 mins until everything is tender. Drain well. Meanwhile, place the salmon fillets in a microwaveable dish, splash with a little water, then cover in cling film and microwave on High for 2½ mins until the fish flakes.
- Heat the grill. Heat the oil in a deep frying pan. Cut the potatoes into chunky slices, then quickly cook in the pan over a high heat until golden on the edges. Flake the salmon into large chunks and poke amongst the potatoes with the broccoli. Stir the mint and some seasoning into the eggs, then pour into the pan. Leave for 6 mins over a low heat until the sides are set and just the centre is a little wobbly, then flash under the grill to set completely and brown. Serve in wedges with a big green salad on the side.

Nutrition Information

- Calories: 440 calories
- Saturated Fat: 6 grams saturated fat
- Total Carbohydrate: 21 grams carbohydrates

10. One Pan Summer Eggs

Serving: 2 | Prep: 5mins | Cook: 12mins | Ready in:

Ingredients

- 1 tbsp olive oil
- 400g courgettes (about 2 large ones), chopped into small chunks
- 200g/7oz pack cherry tomatoes, halved
- 1 garlic clove, crushed
- 2 eggs
- few basil leaves, to serve

Direction

- Heat the oil in a non-stick frying pan, then add the courgettes. Fry for 5 mins, stirring every so often until they start to soften, add the tomatoes and garlic, then cook for a few mins more. Stir in a little seasoning, then make two gaps in the mix and crack in the eggs. Cover the pan with a lid or a sheet of foil, then cook for 2-3 mins until the eggs are done to your liking. Scatter over a few basil leaves and serve with crusty bread.

Nutrition Information

- Calories: 196 calories
- Total Fat: 13 grams fat
- Saturated Fat: 3 grams saturated fat
- Fiber: 3 grams fiber
- Protein: 12 grams protein
- Sodium: 0.25 milligram of sodium
- Sugar: 6 grams sugar
- Total Carbohydrate: 7 grams carbohydrates

11. Orange & Mint Salad

Serving: 4 | Prep: 15mins | Cook: | Ready in:

Ingredients

- 4 oranges
- 12 soft dates, stoned, sliced lengthways
- small bunch mint, leaves finely chopped, plus a few left whole
- 1 tbsp rose syrup or rosewater

Direction

- Peel then segment the oranges, removing the white pith. Place in a bowl along with any juices, then add the dates, chopped mint and rose syrup and toss gently. Divide between 4 dessert bowls, scatter on the mint leaves and serve.

Nutrition Information

- Calories: 222 calories
- Total Carbohydrate: 54 grams carbohydrates
- Sugar: 54 grams sugar
- Fiber: 5 grams fiber
- Protein: 4 grams protein
- Sodium: 0.04 milligram of sodium
- Total Fat: 1 grams fat

12. Oven Baked Egg & Chips

Serving: 2 | Prep: 5mins | Cook: 35mins | Ready in:

Ingredients

- 2 medium baking potatoes, cut into chunky wedges
- 2 tbsp olive oil
- 1 tsp smoked paprika
- 2 tomatoes, halved
- 2 eggs

Direction

- Heat oven to 190C/170C fan/gas 5. Tip the potato wedges into a roasting tin. Drizzle over the oil and sprinkle over the paprika. Season and mix well to coat the potatoes. Roast for 25 mins, turning halfway through, until almost tender.
- Nestle the tomatoes, cut-side up, amongst the potatoes. Make 2 spaces in the tin and crack an egg into each one. Return to the oven for 6-8 mins until the eggs are just set.

Nutrition Information

- Calories: 303 calories
- Protein: 11 grams protein
- Total Fat: 19 grams fat
- Total Carbohydrate: 25 grams carbohydrates
- Fiber: 3 grams fiber
- Sodium: 0.26 milligram of sodium
- Saturated Fat: 3 grams saturated fat
- Sugar: 3 grams sugar

13. Pancetta & Pepper Piperade

Serving: 4 | Prep: 10mins | Cook: 30mins | Ready in:

Ingredients

- 2 x 70g packs pancetta pieces
- 1 red onion, finely chopped
- 3 peppers, 1 each of green, red and yellow, deseeded and finely diced
- 400g can chopped tomatoes
- 2 tbsp tomato purée
- 4 medium eggs
- small handful basil leaves, shredded
- crusty bread, to serve (optional)

Direction

- Put the pancetta and onion in a large, deep frying pan. Cook for 7 mins until the onion is beginning to soften.

- Add the peppers, tomatoes and tomato purée to the pan and mix well. Season, cover and cook for 10-15 mins.
- Make 4 small wells in the mixture. Crack an egg into each well and cook for a further 5-6 mins or until the eggs have set. Scatter with basil and serve straight away, with crusty bread, if you like.

Nutrition Information

- Calories: 259 calories
- Protein: 15 grams protein
- Total Fat: 15 grams fat
- Fiber: 5 grams fiber
- Sugar: 12 grams sugar
- Sodium: 1.3 milligram of sodium
- Saturated Fat: 5 grams saturated fat
- Total Carbohydrate: 13 grams carbohydrates

14. Parsnip Hash Browns

Serving: 6 | Prep: | Cook: | Ready in:

Ingredients

- 450g waxy potato(such as Charlotte)
- 350g parsnipor other root veg
- 1small onion, halved and thinly sliced
- 1 garlic clove, finely chopped
- 1 egg, beaten
- 4-5 tbsp sunflower oil
- 6rashers of streaky baconor slices of prosciutto
- 6stems of cherry tomatoeson the vine
- 6 eggs

Direction

- Peel and coarsely grate the potatoes and parsnips – if you're using a food processor, attach the medium grater. Squeeze out as much liquid as possible with your hands and put them in a bowl.

- Stir in the onion, garlic, egg and season if you like. Divide the mixture into six and roughly shape into flat cakes. Heat 2 tbsp of the oil in a large non-stick frying pan and fry three of the cakes on a low heat for 4-5 mins on each side until golden and tender. Transfer to kitchen paper with a slotted spoon and leave to cool while frying the remainder, adding remaining oil as necessary. Meanwhile grill the bacon and tomatoes, poach the eggs and serve alongside.

Nutrition Information

- Calories: 179 calories
- Sodium: 0.06 milligram of sodium
- Total Fat: 9 grams fat
- Saturated Fat: 1 grams saturated fat
- Total Carbohydrate: 21 grams carbohydrates
- Fiber: 4 grams fiber
- Protein: 4 grams protein

15. Peanut Butter & Banana On Toast

Serving: 1 | Prep: 5mins | Cook: 5mins | Ready in:

Ingredients

- 2 slices granary bread
- 1 small banana
- ½ tsp cinnamon
- 1 tbsp crunchy peanut butter

Direction

- Toast bread and slice banana. Layer banana on one slice of toast and dust with cinnamon. Spread the second slice with peanut butter, then sandwich the two together and eat straight away.

Nutrition Information

- Calories: 307 calories
- Sodium: 1 milligram of sodium
- Sugar: 18 grams sugar
- Total Fat: 9 grams fat
- Saturated Fat: 2 grams saturated fat
- Protein: 11 grams protein
- Total Carbohydrate: 45 grams carbohydrates
- Fiber: 4 grams fiber

16. Seville Orange Marmalade

Serving: Makes 3 x 450g/1lb jars marmalade, plus 1 x 100g/3½oz jar | Prep: | Cook: 2hours | Ready in:

Ingredients

- 4 Seville oranges (about 500g/1lb 2oz in total), scrubbed
- 1.7l water
- 1kg granulated sugar

Direction

- Halve the oranges and squeeze the juice into a large stainless-steel pan. Scoop the pips and pulp into a sieve over the pan and squeeze out as much juice as possible, then tie the pulp and pips in the muslin. Shred the remaining peel and pith, either by hand with a sharp knife or in a food processor (a food processor will give very fine flecks rather than strips of peel). Add the shredded peel and muslin bag to the pan along with the water. Leave to soak overnight. This helps to extract the maximum amount of pectin from the fruit pulp, which will give a better set. It also helps to soften the peel, which will reduce the amount of cooking needed.
- Put the pan over a medium heat, then bring up to a simmer. Cook, uncovered, for 1½-2 hrs, until the peel has become very soft. (The cooking time will be affected by how thickly you have cut the peel.) To see if the peel is ready, pick out a thicker piece and press it between your thumb and finger. It should look slightly see-through and feel soft when you rub it.
- Carefully remove the muslin bag, allow to cool slightly, then, wearing the rubber gloves, squeeze out as much liquid as possible to extract the pectin from the fruit pulp. Discard the bag and weigh the simmered peel mixture. There should be between 775-800g; if less, then top up with water to 775g.
- Put 4 small plates in the freezer, ready to use when testing for setting point. Add the sugar to the pan, then put over a low heat. Warm gently so that the sugar dissolves completely, stirring occasionally. Do not boil, before the sugar is dissolved.
- Increase the heat and bring up to the boil but do not stir while the marmalade is boiling. After about 5 mins the marmalade will start to rise up the pan (it may drop back and then rise again) and larger bubbles will cover the surface. After 8-10 mins boiling, test for setting point. Times will vary according to the size of the pan – in a large pan this takes 7-8 mins, in other pans it may take 12-15 mins. As setting point can be easily missed it's better to test too early than too late.
- To test the setting point: take the pan off the heat and allow the bubbles to subside. Take a plate from the freezer and spoon a little liquid onto the plate, then return to the freezer for 1 min. Push the marmalade along the plate with your finger. If setting point has been reached then the marmalade surface will wrinkle slightly and the marmalade won't run back straight away. If it's not at setting point, return to the heat and boil again for 2 mins before re-testing. Repeat until setting point is reached. If you have a sugar thermometer, setting point is reached at 105C, but it's good to do the plate test as well.
- Leave the marmalade to stand for 10 mins or until starting to thicken. If there's any scum on the surface, spoon it off. Transfer the marmalade to sterilised jars. Cover with a wax disc (wax side down) and seal. When cold, label the jars and store in a cool, dark

cupboard. The marmalade should keep for up to a year.

Nutrition Information

- Calories: 28 calories
- Total Carbohydrate: 7 grams carbohydrates
- Sugar: 7 grams sugar

17. Shakshuka

Serving: 2 | Prep: 5mins | Cook: 20mins | Ready in:

Ingredients

- 1 tbsp olive oil
- 2 red onions, chopped
- 1 red chilli, deseeded and finely chopped
- 1 garlic clove, sliced
- small bunch coriander stalks and leaves chopped separately
- 2 cans cherry tomatoes
- 1 tsp caster sugar
- 4 eggs

Direction

- Heat the oil in a frying pan that has a lid, then soften the onions, chilli, garlic and coriander stalks for 5 mins until soft. Stir in the tomatoes and sugar, then bubble for 8-10 mins until thick. Can be frozen for 1 month.
- Using the back of a large spoon, make 4 dips in the sauce, then crack an egg into each one. Put a lid on the pan, then cook over a low heat for 6-8 mins, until the eggs are done to your liking. Scatter with the coriander leaves and serve with crusty bread.

Nutrition Information

- Calories: 340 calories
- Total Fat: 20 grams fat
- Saturated Fat: 5 grams saturated fat

- Total Carbohydrate: 21 grams carbohydrates
- Sugar: 17 grams sugar
- Protein: 21 grams protein
- Sodium: 1.25 milligram of sodium

18. Soft Boiled Egg, Bacon & Watercress Salad

Serving: 2 | Prep: 10mins | Cook: 5mins | Ready in:

Ingredients

- 2 large eggs, at room temperature
- 1 shallot, very finely chopped
- 1 tbsp red wine vinegar
- 1 heaped tsp wholegrain mustard
- 2 tbsp rapeseed oil
- handful chives, snipped (optional)
- 4 thick rashers streaky smoked dry-cured bacon
- 2 slices good white crusty bread(ideally sourdough)
- 2 good handfuls British watercress, thick stems removed

Direction

- Put the eggs in a pan of cold water and bring to the boil. Boil for 3 mins, then lift into a bowl of iced water and cool completely. Very carefully peel away the shells. Leave the eggs in the iced water until you finish the recipe, or for up to 1 hr ahead.
- Mix the shallot with the vinegar and a pinch of salt, then set aside for a few minutes to soften. Whisk in the mustard, oil and chives, if using, to make a dressing.
- Heat the grill to low-medium and cook the bacon until crisp right through. Remove the bacon, then brush the bacon juice and fat all over the bread. Grill the bread for about 1 min on each side until crisp, then cut into soldiers and keep warm.
- Just before serving, bring the pan of water back to the boil and add the eggs. Boil for 1

min to reheat. Toss the dressing with the watercress and divide between 2 plates. Top with an egg and 2 rashers of bacon, with the toast to the side. The egg yolks will still be runny inside.

Nutrition Information

- Calories: 438 calories
- Sodium: 3.3 milligram of sodium
- Total Fat: 28 grams fat
- Saturated Fat: 6 grams saturated fat
- Total Carbohydrate: 26 grams carbohydrates
- Sugar: 1 grams sugar
- Protein: 21 grams protein
- Fiber: 2 grams fiber

19. The Ultimate Makeover: Full English Breakfast

Serving: 2 | Prep: | Cook: 20mins | Ready in:

Ingredients

- 4 rashers good-quality lean unsmoked back bacon
- 4 brown-cap portabello mushrooms
- 12-16 cherry tomatoes on the vine, room temperature
- 6 tsp olive oil
- 2 slices granary or wholegrain bread, cut on the diagonal
- 2 good-quality free-range pork sausages, minimum 86% pork
- 2 free-range, omega-3 rich eggs, room temperature
- few drops cider vinegar
- 2 x 100ml / 3.5 fl oz glasses freshly-squeezed orange juice, plus 1 orange cut into wedges
- handful fresh blueberries (about 50g/2oz)

Direction

- Lay the bacon, mushrooms and tomatoes on a foil-lined tray. Brush the tops of the mushrooms with 3 tsp of the oil and both sides of the bread with the remaining oil. Set aside. Heat the grill to very hot. Lay the sausages on a small foil-lined tray (best not to prick good-quality sausages or they may lose moisture). Grill for about 10 mins until cooked, turning occasionally.
- Meanwhile, three-quarters fill a small pan, and a wide, deep sauté pan with water. Bring both to the boil. Lower an egg into the small pan and remove after 30 secs. Crack the egg into a cup. Add vinegar to the larger pan then, using a wire whisk, swirl the water around to create a whirlpool. Remove the whisk and slowly tip the egg into the centre of the whirlpool (see top picture). When the water comes back to the boil, remove the pan from the heat, cover and leave for 3 mins, then remove the egg. Place in a bowl of warm water while you cook the other egg – or cook both eggs an hour ahead, leave in a bowl of iced water, then reheat for 1½ mins in simmering water before serving.
- Meanwhile heat a griddle pan to very hot. Place the tomatoes, bacon and mushrooms under the grill for 3-4 mins without turning. At the same time, lay the bread on the griddle pan, cook until crisp, about 1 min each side. Drain everything on kitchen paper.
- Remove the eggs with a slotted spoon and drain briefly on a cloth. Arrange everything on a plate and serve with the juice and fruit.

Nutrition Information

- Calories: 618 calories
- Protein: 37 grams protein
- Total Fat: 37 grams fat
- Sugar: 21 grams sugar
- Fiber: 5 grams fiber
- Total Carbohydrate: 37 grams carbohydrates
- Saturated Fat: 11 grams saturated fat
- Sodium: 3.05 milligram of sodium

20. Tropical Breakfast Smoothie

Serving: 3 | Prep: 5mins | Cook: | Ready in:

Ingredients

- 3 passion fruits
- 1 banana, chopped
- 1small mango, peeled, stoned and chopped
- 300ml orange juice
- ice cubes

Direction

- Scoop the pulp of the passion fruits into a blender and add the banana, mango and orange juice. Purée until smooth and drink immediately, topped with ice cubes.

Nutrition Information

- Calories: 189 calories
- Saturated Fat: 0.1 grams saturated fat
- Protein: 4 grams protein
- Fiber: 10 grams fiber
- Total Fat: 1 grams fat
- Total Carbohydrate: 37 grams carbohydrates
- Sugar: 35 grams sugar
- Sodium: 0.1 milligram of sodium

21. Vegan Tomato & Mushroom Pancakes

Serving: 2 | Prep: 5mins | Cook: 30mins | Ready in:

Ingredients

- 140g white self-raising flour
- 1 tsp soya flour
- 400ml soya milk
- vegetable oil, for frying
- For the topping
- 2 tbsp vegetable oil
- 250g button mushrooms
- 250g cherry tomatoes, halved
- 2 tbsp soya cream or soya milk
- large handful pine nuts
- snipped chives, to serve

Direction

- Sift the flours and a pinch of salt into a blender. Add the soya milk and blend to make a smooth batter.
- Heat a little oil in a medium non-stick frying pan until very hot. Pour about 3 tbsp of the batter into the pan and cook over a medium heat until bubbles appear on the surface of the pancake. Flip the pancake over with a palette knife and cook the other side until golden brown. Repeat with the remaining batter, keeping the cooked pancakes warm as you go. You will make about 8.
- For the topping, heat the oil in a frying pan. Cook the mushrooms until tender, add the tomatoes and cook for a couple of mins. Pour in the soya cream or milk and pine nuts, then gently cook until combined. Divide the pancakes between 2 plates, then spoon over the tomatoes and mushrooms. Scatter with chives.

Nutrition Information

- Calories: 609 calories
- Total Carbohydrate: 59 grams carbohydrates
- Saturated Fat: 4 grams saturated fat
- Fiber: 6 grams fiber
- Protein: 18 grams protein
- Sugar: 6 grams sugar
- Sodium: 0.87 milligram of sodium
- Total Fat: 35 grams fat

Chapter 2: Dairy-Free Lucnh Recipes

***

22. Barbecued Fennel With Black Olive Dressing

Serving: 4 | Prep: 10mins | Cook: 10mins | Ready in:

Ingredients

- 2 fennel bulbs, sliced lengthways into 1cm-thick pieces
- 1 ½ tbsp olive oil
- 2 tbsp finely chopped black Kalamata olive
- 1 garlic clove, crushed
- juice 1 lemon
- small handful each parsley and basil, finely chopped

Direction

- Heat a BBQ or griddle pan. Toss the fennel in 1 tbsp of the oil, coating well. Cook for 5 mins on each side until golden brown and charred.
- To make the dressing, put the olives, garlic, lemon juice and remaining oil in a bowl. Add the chopped herbs and combine. Lay the fennel on a platter and pour over the dressing. Eat warm or at room temperature.

Nutrition Information

- Calories: 69 calories
- Sugar: 2 grams sugar
- Total Fat: 6 grams fat
- Protein: 1 grams protein
- Sodium: 0.2 milligram of sodium
- Fiber: 5 grams fiber
- Total Carbohydrate: 3 grams carbohydrates
- Saturated Fat: 1 grams saturated fat

23. Crunchy Prawn & Noodle Salad

Serving: 2 | Prep: 15mins | Cook: | Ready in:

Ingredients

- 100g rice noodle
- 2 small carrots, cut into thin matchsticks
- 2 spring onions, thinly sliced
- small handful each coriander and mint, chopped
- 140g cooked prawn in chilli, lime and coriander (we used Waitrose)
- 2 tsp reduced-salt soy sauce
- 1 tsp fish sauce
- 2 tsp light soft brown sugar
- zest and juice 1 lime

Direction

- Soak the noodles in boiling water following the pack instructions. Drain and run under cold water until cool, then drain well again. Mix the noodles with the carrots, spring onions, coriander, mint and prawns.
- In a small bowl, whisk the remaining ingredients together, pour over the noodle salad and toss well to coat. Store in containers until ready to eat.

Nutrition Information

- Calories: 316 calories
- Protein: 18 grams protein
- Sodium: 1.9 milligram of sodium
- Total Fat: 2 grams fat
- Total Carbohydrate: 51 grams carbohydrates
- Sugar: 12 grams sugar
- Fiber: 4 grams fiber

24. Curried Squash, Lentil & Coconut Soup

Serving: 6 | Prep: 10mins | Cook: 25mins | Ready in:

Ingredients

- 1 tbsp olive oil
- 1 butternut squash, peeled, deseeded and diced
- 200g carrot, diced
- 1 tbsp curry powder containing turmeric
- 100g red lentil
- 700ml low-sodium vegetable stock
- 1 can reduced-fat coconut milk
- coriander and naan bread, to serve

Direction

- Heat the oil in a large saucepan, add the squash and carrots, sizzle for 1 min, then stir in the curry powder and cook for 1 min more. Tip in the lentils, the vegetable stock and coconut milk and give everything a good stir. Bring to the boil, then turn the heat down and simmer for 15-18 mins until everything is tender.
- Using a hand blender or in a food processor, blitz until as smooth as you like. Season and serve scattered with roughly chopped coriander and some naan bread alongside.

Nutrition Information

- Calories: 178 calories
- Total Carbohydrate: 22 grams carbohydrates
- Sugar: 9 grams sugar
- Fiber: 4 grams fiber
- Protein: 6 grams protein
- Total Fat: 7 grams fat
- Saturated Fat: 5 grams saturated fat
- Sodium: 0.4 milligram of sodium

25. Egg & Rocket Pizzas

Serving: 2 | Prep: 10mins | Cook: 20mins | Ready in:

Ingredients

- 2 seeded wraps
- a little olive oil, for brushing
- 1 roasted red pepper, from a jar
- 2 tomatoes
- 2 tbsp tomato purée
- 1 tbsp chopped dill
- 2 tbsp chopped parsley
- 2 eggs
- 65g pack rocket
- ½ red onion, very thinly sliced

Direction

- Heat oven to 200C/180C fan/gas 6. Lay the tortillas on two baking sheets, brush sparingly with the oil then bake for 3 mins. Meanwhile chop the pepper and tomatoes and mix with the tomato purée, seasoning and herbs. Turn the tortillas over and spread with the tomato mixture, leaving the centre free from any large pieces of pepper or tomato.
- Break an egg into the centre then return to the oven for 10 mins or until the egg is just set and the tortilla is crispy round the edges. Serve scattered with the rocket and onion.

Nutrition Information

- Calories: 327 calories
- Sugar: 8 grams sugar
- Sodium: 1 milligram of sodium
- Total Carbohydrate: 39 grams carbohydrates
- Fiber: 5 grams fiber
- Total Fat: 11 grams fat
- Saturated Fat: 3 grams saturated fat
- Protein: 15 grams protein

26. Herby Celery & Bulgur Salad

Serving: 6 | Prep: 30mins | Cook: | Ready in:

Ingredients

- 200g bulgur wheat
- 1 bunch celery

- 1 dessert apple
- juice 1 lemon
- 4 tbsp olive oil
- handful toasted hazelnuts, roughly chopped
- 1 red chilli, deseeded and chopped
- large handful pomegranate seeds
- small bunch parsley, chopped
- small bunch mint, chopped
- small bunch tarragon, chopped

Direction

- Put the bulgur wheat in a large bowl and just cover with boiling water. Cover the bowl with cling film and leave for 30 mins to absorb all the water.
- Meanwhile, separate the sticks of celery and set the leaves aside. Very finely slice the celery and roughly chop the leaves. Cut the apple into fine matchsticks and toss in a little lemon juice. In a bowl, mix the remaining lemon juice with the oil and some seasoning to make a dressing.
- Gently fluff up the bulgur with a fork. Mix the sliced celery and apple through the bulgur, followed by the nuts, chilli, pomegranate seeds and herbs. Drizzle over the dressing and toss everything together gently. Scatter with the celery leaves and serve.

Nutrition Information

- Calories: 229 calories
- Total Carbohydrate: 30 grams carbohydrates
- Sodium: 0.1 milligram of sodium
- Saturated Fat: 1 grams saturated fat
- Fiber: 2 grams fiber
- Sugar: 5 grams sugar
- Protein: 4 grams protein
- Total Fat: 10 grams fat

27. Jewelled Couscous

Serving: 10 | Prep: 12mins | Cook: | Ready in:

Ingredients

- 400g couscous
- 2 tbsp lemon-infused oil
- 500g soft dried apricot, chopped
- 1 cucumber, deseeded and chopped
- 1 large yellow pepper, deseeded and chopped
- 140g pitted black olive, chopped
- 140g sundried tomato, chopped
- small bunch parsley, chopped
- 12 cherry tomatoes, halved

Direction

- Place the couscous in a bowl and cover with 700ml boiling water. Cover with cling film and leave for 10 mins, until all the liquid has been absorbed.
- Pour over the oil and some seasoning, mix and fluff up the couscous with a fork.
- Gently stir through the remaining ingredients and serve.

Nutrition Information

- Calories: 249 calories
- Total Fat: 7 grams fat
- Saturated Fat: 1 grams saturated fat
- Total Carbohydrate: 40 grams carbohydrates
- Sugar: 20 grams sugar
- Fiber: 6 grams fiber
- Protein: 6 grams protein
- Sodium: 0.7 milligram of sodium

28. Kale & Apple Soup With Walnuts

Serving: 2 | Prep: 20mins | Cook: 15mins | Ready in:

Ingredients

- 8 walnut halves, broken into pieces
- 1 onion, finely chopped
- 2 carrots, coarsely grated

- 2 red apples, unpeeled and finely chopped
- 1 tbsp cider vinegar
- 500ml reduced-salt vegetable stock
- 200g kale, roughly chopped
- 20g pack of dried apple crisps (optional)

Direction

- In a dry, non-stick frying pan, cook the walnut pieces for 2-3 mins until toasted, turning frequently so they don't burn. Take off the heat and allow to cool.
- Put the onion, carrots, apples, vinegar and stock in a large saucepan and bring to the boil. Reduce the heat and simmer for 10 mins, stirring occasionally.
- Once the onion is translucent and the apples start to soften, add the kale and simmer for an additional 2 mins. Carefully transfer to a blender or liquidiser and blend until very smooth. Pour into bowls and serve topped with the toasted walnuts, and a sprinkling of apple crisps, if you like.

Nutrition Information

- Calories: 403 calories
- Total Fat: 21 grams fat
- Saturated Fat: 2 grams saturated fat
- Total Carbohydrate: 36 grams carbohydrates
- Sodium: 0.8 milligram of sodium
- Sugar: 25 grams sugar
- Fiber: 9 grams fiber
- Protein: 12 grams protein

29. Mediterranean Potato Salad

Serving: 4 | Prep: 10mins | Cook: 25mins | Ready in:

Ingredients

- 1 tbsp olive oil
- 1 small onion, thinly sliced
- 1 garlic clove, crushed

- 1 tsp oregano, fresh or dried
- ½ x 400g can cherry tomatoes
- 100g roasted red pepper, from a jar, sliced
- 300g new potato, halved if large
- 25g black olive, sliced
- handful basil leaves, torn

Direction

- Heat the oil in a saucepan, add the onion and cook for 5-10 mins until soft. Add the garlic and oregano and cook for 1 min. Add the tomatoes and peppers, season well and simmer gently for 10 mins.
- Meanwhile, cook the potatoes in a pan of boiling salted water for 10-15 mins until tender. Drain well, mix with the sauce and serve warm, sprinkled with olives and basil.

Nutrition Information

- Calories: 111 calories
- Sodium: 0.2 milligram of sodium
- Fiber: 2 grams fiber
- Protein: 3 grams protein
- Total Carbohydrate: 16 grams carbohydrates
- Total Fat: 4 grams fat
- Sugar: 3 grams sugar
- Saturated Fat: 1 grams saturated fat

30. Minestrone Soup

Serving: 4 | Prep: 15mins | Cook: 30mins | Ready in:

Ingredients

- 3 large carrots, roughly chopped
- 1 large onion, roughly chopped
- 4 celery sticks, roughly chopped
- 1 tbsp olive oil
- 2 garlic cloves, crushed
- 2 large potatoes, cut into small dice
- 2 tbsp tomato purée
- 2l vegetable stock

- 400g can chopped tomatoes
- 400g can butter or cannellini beans
- 140g spaghetti, snapped into short lengths
- ½ head Savoy cabbage, shredded
- crusty bread, to serve

Direction

- In a food processor, whizz the carrots, onion and celery into small pieces. Heat the oil in a pan, add the processed vegetables, garlic and potatoes, then cook over a high heat for 5 mins until softened.
- Stir in the tomato purée, stock and tomatoes. Bring to the boil, then turn down the heat and simmer, covered, for 10 mins.
- Tip in the beans and pasta, then cook for a further 10 mins, adding the cabbage for the final 2 mins. Season to taste and serve with crusty bread.

Nutrition Information

- Calories: 420 calories
- Sugar: 24 grams sugar
- Fiber: 16 grams fiber
- Sodium: 1.11 milligram of sodium
- Total Fat: 6 grams fat
- Protein: 18 grams protein
- Total Carbohydrate: 79 grams carbohydrates
- Saturated Fat: 1 grams saturated fat

31. Miso Prawn Skewers With Veggie Rice Salad

Serving: 4 | Prep: 15mins | Cook: 25mins | Ready in:

Ingredients

- 200g brown basmati rice
- 175g mange tout
- 200g frozen soy bean
- 1 ½ tbsp sesame oil
- 4 spring onions, finely sliced

- large handful coriander, roughly chopped
- 1 green chilli, finely diced
- For the skewers
- 400g raw large peeled prawn
- 3 tbsp sweet miso paste (You'll find this with the Japanese ingredients. We used Clearspring white miso)
- 2 tsp soy sauce
- 2 tsp Japanese rice vinegar
- 2 tsp soft brown sugar

Direction

- Place the brown rice in a pan with lots of cold water. Bring to the boil and simmer for 20-25 mins or until tender. Meanwhile, soak wooden skewers in some cold water (to prevent them burning). Add the mangetout and soy beans to the rice for the final 5 mins of cooking. Rinse under cold water, draining thoroughly.
- Toss the rice with the sesame oil and mix in a large bowl with the spring onions, coriander, chilli and seasoning.
- Heat a grill. Place the skewer ingredients in a bowl with a few grinds of black pepper. Give everything a good stir, making sure the prawns are well coated. Thread prawns onto the skewers and lay on a baking sheet. Grill for a couple of mins each side, turning, until prawns are cooked through. Serve with the rice salad and drizzle over any of the cooking juices.

Nutrition Information

- Calories: 410 calories
- Sugar: 8 grams sugar
- Protein: 32 grams protein
- Sodium: 1.5 milligram of sodium
- Total Fat: 10 grams fat
- Saturated Fat: 2 grams saturated fat
- Total Carbohydrate: 47 grams carbohydrates
- Fiber: 7 grams fiber

32. Miso Steak

Serving: 2 | Prep: 10mins | Cook: 10mins | Ready in:

Ingredients

- 2 tbsp brown miso paste
- 1 tbsp dry sherry or sake
- 1 tbsp caster sugar
- 2 crushed garlic cloves
- 300g/11oz lean steak
- baby spinach, sliced cucumber, celery, radish and toasted sesame seeds, to serve

Direction

- Tip the miso paste, Sherry or sake, sugar and garlic into a sealable food bag. Season with a generous grinding of black pepper, then squash it all together until completely mixed. Add the steak, gently massage the marinade into the steak until completely coated, then seal the bag. Pop the bag into the fridge and leave for at least 1 hr, but up to 2 days is fine.
- To cook, heat a heavy-based frying pan, griddle pan or barbecue until very hot. Wipe the excess marinade off the steak, then sear for 3 mins on each side for medium-rare or a few mins longer if you prefer the meat more cooked. Set aside for 1 min to rest. Carve the beef into thick slices and serve with a crunchy salad made with the spinach, cucumber, celery, radish and sesame seeds.

Nutrition Information

- Calories: 232 calories
- Total Carbohydrate: 4 grams carbohydrates
- Sugar: 3 grams sugar
- Protein: 32 grams protein
- Sodium: 0.66 milligram of sodium
- Total Fat: 9 grams fat
- Saturated Fat: 4 grams saturated fat

33. Mixed Bean & Wild Rice Salad

Serving: 8 | Prep: 10mins | Cook: 25mins | Ready in:

Ingredients

- 375g rice mix, we used brown basmati & wild rice
- 2 x 400g cans mixed beans, drained and rinsed
- 340g can sweetcorn, drained
- 1 small red onion, finely sliced
- 2 red peppers, deseeded and diced
- zest and juice 1 lime
- 2 tsp honey
- 1 red chilli, deseeded and finely sliced
- small bunch coriander, leaves picked

Direction

- Cook rice following pack instructions. Once cooked, rinse under cold water to cool down. Once cold combine in a bowl with the beans, sweetcorn, onion and red peppers.
- Mix the lime zest and juice, honey and chilli. Pour over the rice mixture and mix well, then season to taste. Stir through the coriander leaves just before serving.

Nutrition Information

- Calories: 367 calories
- Sugar: 11 grams sugar
- Fiber: 8 grams fiber
- Protein: 12 grams protein
- Sodium: 1.2 milligram of sodium
- Total Fat: 2 grams fat
- Total Carbohydrate: 74 grams carbohydrates

34. Moroccan Turkey Salad

Serving: 4 | Prep: 20mins | Cook: 15mins | Ready in:

Ingredients

- 2 pitta breads

- 2 tbsp olive oil
- 1 diced aubergine
- 1 tbsp harissa
- 250g halved cherry tomato
- 500g shredded leftover turkeybreast
- 100g rocket
- seeds 1 pomegranateor 110g tub pomegranate seeds
- a few mintleaves

Direction

- Tear the pitta into pieces and fry in the olive oil until crisp. Tip into a bowl, then fry the aubergine for 10 mins until soft. Add to the pitta with the harissa, tomatoes, turkey and rocket. Toss well. Scatter over pomegranate seeds and mint leaves.

Nutrition Information

- Calories: 360 calories
- Protein: 47 grams protein
- Total Carbohydrate: 22 grams carbohydrates
- Fiber: 4 grams fiber
- Sodium: 0.6 milligram of sodium
- Total Fat: 9 grams fat
- Saturated Fat: 2 grams saturated fat
- Sugar: 6 grams sugar

35. Pasta Salad With Tuna, Capers & Balsamic Dressing

Serving: 4 | Prep: 10mins | Cook: 10mins | Ready in:

Ingredients

- 350g orecchiette pasta
- 225g jar MSC approved tuna in spring water, drained
- 1 tbsp caper, drained
- 15 peppadew peppers from a jar, chopped
- 1 celery heart, sliced

- 140g yellow, red or a mixture of cherry tomato, halved
- 75ml balsamic vinegar
- 3 tbsp extra-virgin olive oil
- 100g bag rocket leaves
- good handful basil leaves

Direction

- Cook the pasta following pack instructions, then drain and rinse in cold water. After draining again, transfer to a large bowl. Add the remaining ingredients except the basil, season well, and toss to combine. Scatter with basil and serve.

Nutrition Information

- Calories: 527 calories
- Saturated Fat: 2 grams saturated fat
- Protein: 24 grams protein
- Total Fat: 10 grams fat
- Sugar: 16 grams sugar
- Fiber: 3 grams fiber
- Sodium: 0.6 milligram of sodium
- Total Carbohydrate: 82 grams carbohydrates

36. Pasta With Pine Nuts, Broccoli, Sardines & Fennel

Serving: 6 | Prep: 15mins | Cook: 15mins | Ready in:

Ingredients

- 4 tbsp extra-virgin olive oil, plus a splash
- 500g bucatini or long pasta, like spaghetti
- 500g purple sprouting broccoli, stalks halved if very large
- 2 red onions, sliced
- 4 garlic cloves, thinly sliced
- 1 small fennel bulb, very thinly sliced
- 50g salted sardine, or good-quality canned sardines in oil
- 25g pine nut

- 25g raisin
- juice and zest ½ lemon
- chilli flakes

Direction

- Bring a large pan of water to the boil, with a splash of oil, then add the pasta. Cook following pack instructions, adding the broccoli for the final 5 mins.
- Meanwhile, gently heat the oil in a large pan. Add the onions and sliced garlic, and cook slowly for 2 mins. Add the fennel and cook for a couple more mins, until softened. Flake the sardines into the pan and stir around for a few more mins to break them up.
- Tip the pasta and broccoli into the pan with the pine nuts, raisins and lemon juice. Toss together to let the pasta absorb the oil, season well and serve immediately, scattered with lemon zest and chilli flakes.

Nutrition Information

- Calories: 462 calories
- Fiber: 7 grams fiber
- Saturated Fat: 2 grams saturated fat
- Protein: 18 grams protein
- Total Carbohydrate: 67 grams carbohydrates
- Sugar: 10 grams sugar
- Sodium: 0.1 milligram of sodium
- Total Fat: 13 grams fat

37. Prawn & Pink Grapefruit Noodle Salad

Serving: 6 | Prep: 25mins | Cook: | Ready in:

Ingredients

- 200g thin rice noodle (vermicelli)
- 12 cherry tomatoes, halved
- 1 tbsp fish sauce
- juice 1 lime
- 2 tsp palm sugar or soft brown sugar
- 1 large red chilli, ½ diced, ½ sliced
- 2 pink grapefruits, segmented
- ½ cucumber, peeled, deseeded and thinly sliced
- 2 carrots, cut into matchsticks
- 3 spring onions, thinly sliced
- 400g cooked large prawn
- large handful mint, leaves picked
- large handful coriander, leaves picked

Direction

- Put the noodles in a bowl, breaking them up a little, and cover with boiling water from the kettle. Leave to soak for 10 mins until tender. Drain, rinse under cold running water, then leave the noodles to drain thoroughly.
- In the same bowl, lightly squash the cherry tomatoes – we used the end of a rolling pin. Stir in the fish sauce, lime juice, sugar and diced chilli. Taste for the right balance of sweet, sour and spicy – adjust if necessary (see tip, below).
- Toss through the noodles, then add all the remaining ingredients, except the sliced chilli. Season and give everything a good stir, then divide the noodle salad between 6 serving dishes and sprinkle over the chilli before serving.

Nutrition Information

- Calories: 228 calories
- Sugar: 6 grams sugar
- Fiber: 2 grams fiber
- Protein: 13 grams protein
- Sodium: 1.6 milligram of sodium
- Total Fat: 1 grams fat
- Total Carbohydrate: 38 grams carbohydrates

38. Prawn, Pomegranate & Grapefruit Salad

Serving: 6 | Prep: 20mins | Cook: | Ready in:

Ingredients

- 2 pink grapefruits, zest and juice from 1, segments cut from the other
- 2 tbsp olive oil
- 1 tbsp red wine vinegar
- 1 tsp caster sugar
- 2 tbsp chopped dill
- 300g cooked, peeled prawn
- ½ cucumber, halved lengthways, seeds scooped out with a teaspoon, diced
- 2 shallots, finely chopped
- 2 handfuls frisée, torn
- 2 handfuls rocket
- 100g pack pomegranate seeds

Direction

- Whisk together the grapefruit zest and juice, oil, vinegar, sugar and dill to make a dressing. Mix half with the prawns and allow to marinate for 10 mins.
- Just before serving, gently toss the cucumber, shallots, frisée and rocket with the remaining dressing. Add a pile to each of 6 starter plates, along with the prawns and grapefruit segments. Scatter over the pomegranate seeds and serve.

Nutrition Information

- Calories: 113 calories
- Sodium: 0.8 milligram of sodium
- Total Fat: 4 grams fat
- Saturated Fat: 1 grams saturated fat
- Protein: 9 grams protein
- Total Carbohydrate: 10 grams carbohydrates
- Sugar: 4 grams sugar
- Fiber: 1 grams fiber

39. Quinoa Tabbouleh

Serving: 2 | Prep: 20mins | Cook: 20mins | Ready in:

Ingredients

- 100g dried quinoa
- 75g parsley, roughly chopped
- 300g tomatoes, cut into 1cm dice (no need to remove the seeds)
- 100g cucumber, cut into small dice
- For the dressing
- 1 tbsp olive oil
- 2 tbsp balsamic vinegar
- juice and zest 0.5 lemon
- drop of vanilla extract
- 1 tsp rice syrup or agave
- pinch of Himalayan pink salt
- ½ garlic clove, crushed
- 50g salad leaves, to serve

Direction

- Cook the quinoa following pack instructions, then set aside to cool.
- Make the dressing by adding the olive oil, vinegar, lemon juice, vanilla extract, rice syrup, pinch of salt and garlic into a jug and whisk until smooth. Mix this into the quinoa and mix together with all the other ingredients. Serve on a bed of salad leaves.

Nutrition Information

- Calories: 284 calories
- Saturated Fat: 1 grams saturated fat
- Fiber: 5 grams fiber
- Sugar: 14 grams sugar
- Protein: 10 grams protein
- Sodium: 0.4 milligram of sodium
- Total Fat: 9 grams fat
- Total Carbohydrate: 38 grams carbohydrates

40. Spiced Carrot & Lentil Soup

Serving: 4 | Prep: 10mins | Cook: 15mins | Ready in:

Ingredients

- 2 tsp cumin seeds
- pinch chilli flakes
- 2 tbsp olive oil
- 600g carrots, washed and coarsely grated (no need to peel)
- 140g split red lentils
- 1l hot vegetable stock (from a cube is fine)
- 125ml milk (to make it dairy-free, see 'try' below)
- plain yogurt and naan bread, to serve

Direction

- Heat a large saucepan and dry-fry 2 tsp cumin seeds and a pinch of chilli flakes for 1 min, or until they start to jump around the pan and release their aromas.
- Scoop out about half with a spoon and set aside. Add 2 tbsp olive oil, 600g coarsely grated carrots, 140g split red lentils, 1l hot vegetable stock and 125ml milk to the pan and bring to the boil.
- Simmer for 15 mins until the lentils have swollen and softened.
- Whizz the soup with a stick blender or in a food processor until smooth (or leave it chunky if you prefer).
- Season to taste and finish with a dollop of plain yogurt and a sprinkling of the reserved toasted spices. Serve with warmed naan breads.

Nutrition Information

- Calories: 238 calories
- Protein: 11 grams protein
- Sodium: 0.25 milligram of sodium
- Total Fat: 7 grams fat
- Saturated Fat: 1 grams saturated fat
- Total Carbohydrate: 34 grams carbohydrates
- Fiber: 5 grams fiber

41. Spiced Cauliflower With Chickpeas, Herbs & Pine Nuts

Serving: 4 | Prep: 10mins | Cook: 40mins | Ready in:

Ingredients

- 1 large head cauliflower, broken into florets (about 1kg in total)
- 2 garlic cloves, crushed
- 2 tsp each caraway and cumin seed
- 3 tbsp olive oil
- 400g can chickpea, drained and rinsed
- 100g pine nut
- small bunch each parsley and dill, leaves torn

Direction

- Heat oven to 200C/180C fan/gas 6. Toss the cauliflower, garlic, spices, 2 tbsp oil and some seasoning in a roasting tin, then roast for 30 mins.
- Add the chickpeas, pine nuts and remaining oil to the tin, then cook for 10 mins more. To serve, stir in the herbs with your chosen dressing.

Nutrition Information

- Calories: 407 calories
- Fiber: 10 grams fiber
- Protein: 17 grams protein
- Saturated Fat: 3 grams saturated fat
- Total Fat: 29 grams fat
- Sugar: 7 grams sugar
- Total Carbohydrate: 19 grams carbohydrates
- Sodium: 0.5 milligram of sodium

42. Spiced Vegetable Pilaf

Serving: 4 | Prep: 10mins | Cook: 40mins | Ready in:

Ingredients

- 6 carrots, cut lengthways into 6-8 wedges
- 3 red onions, cut into wedges
- 2 tbsp olive oil
- 2 tsp cumin seeds
- 4 cardamom pods
- 1 cinnamon stick
- 200g brown basmati rice, rinsed
- 400ml vegetable stock
- 400g can brown lentils, rinsed and drained
- 200g baby spinach
- handful toasted flaked almonds, or a few whole almonds (optional)

Direction

- Heat oven to 200C/180C fan/gas 6. In boiling water, cook carrots for 4 mins, tipping in onions for the last min of cooking. Drain and mix in a roasting tin with 4 tsp oil, the cumin and seasoning. Roast for 30 mins, while you cook the rice.
- Heat remaining 2 tsp oil in a large pan. Add cardamom and cinnamon for 30 secs, then add rice and toast for 1 min. Pour over stock and 100ml water, then simmer, covered, for 25-30 mins, until rice is tender and the water absorbed. Remove cinnamon and cardamom.
- Tip in lentils and fork through before topping with spinach. Put lid back on and cook over a low heat, stirring once, until spinach has wilted and lentils heated through. Fork through again before tipping the cumin roasted veg onto the top and sprinkling with almonds, if using.

Nutrition Information

- Calories: 375 calories
- Sodium: 0.6 milligram of sodium
- Sugar: 18 grams sugar
- Total Fat: 9 grams fat
- Fiber: 11 grams fiber
- Protein: 12 grams protein
- Saturated Fat: 1 grams saturated fat
- Total Carbohydrate: 66 grams carbohydrates

43. Spicy Chicken & Avocado Wraps

Serving: 2 | Prep: 5mins | Cook: 8mins | Ready in:

Ingredients

- 1 chicken breast (approx 180g), thinly sliced at an angle
- generous squeeze juice 0.5 lime
- ½ tsp mild chilli powder
- 1 garlic clove, chopped
- 1 tsp olive oil
- 2 seeded wraps
- 1 avocado, halved and stoned
- 1 roasted red pepper from a jar, sliced
- a few sprigs coriander, chopped

Direction

- Mix the chicken with the lime juice, chilli powder and garlic.
- Heat the oil in a non-stick frying pan then fry the chicken for a couple of mins – it will cook very quickly so keep an eye on it. Meanwhile, warm the wraps following the pack instructions or, if you have a gas hob, heat them over the flame to slightly char them. Do not let them dry out or they are difficult to roll.
- Squash half an avocado onto each wrap, add the peppers to the pan to warm them through then pile onto the wraps with the chicken, and sprinkle over the coriander. Roll up, cut in half and eat with your fingers.

Nutrition Information

- Calories: 403 calories
- Total Carbohydrate: 32 grams carbohydrates

- Fiber: 5 grams fiber
- Sodium: 0.8 milligram of sodium
- Sugar: 2 grams sugar
- Protein: 29 grams protein
- Total Fat: 16 grams fat
- Saturated Fat: 4 grams saturated fat

44. Squash & Barley Salad With Balsamic Vinaigrette

Serving: 8 | Prep: | Cook: 25mins | Ready in:

Ingredients

- 1 butternut squash, peeled and cut into long pieces
- 1 tbsp olive oil
- 250g pearl barley
- 300g Tenderstem broccoli, cut into medium-size pieces
- 100g SunBlush tomato, sliced
- 1 small red onion, diced
- 2 tbsp pumpkin seeds
- 1 tbsp small capers, rinsed
- 15 black olives, pitted
- 20g pack basil, chopped
- For the dressing
- 5 tbsp balsamic vinegar
- 6 tbsp extra-virgin olive oil
- 1 tbsp Dijon mustard
- 1 garlic clove, finely chopped

Direction

- Heat oven to 200C/fan 180C/gas 6. Place the squash on a baking tray and toss with olive oil. Roast for 20 mins. Meanwhile, boil the barley for about 25 mins in salted water until tender, but al dente. While this is happening, whisk the dressing ingredients in a small bowl, then season with salt and pepper. Drain the barley, then tip it into a bowl and pour over the dressing. Mix well and let it cool.
- Boil the broccoli in salted water until just tender, then drain and rinse in cold water.

Drain and pat dry. Add the broccoli and remaining ingredients to the barley and mix well. This will keep for 3 days in the fridge and is delicious warm or cold.

Nutrition Information

- Calories: 301 calories
- Protein: 6 grams protein
- Sodium: 0.55 milligram of sodium
- Total Fat: 14 grams fat
- Saturated Fat: 2 grams saturated fat
- Total Carbohydrate: 40 grams carbohydrates
- Sugar: 9 grams sugar

45. Squash, Orange & Barley Salad

Serving: 6 | Prep: 40mins | Cook: 40mins | Ready in:

Ingredients

- 175g pearl barley
- 1kg peeled squash or 1 butternut squash, unpeeled
- 3 tbsp olive oil
- zest and juice 1 orange
- 4 tbsp red wine vinegar
- ½ red onion, thinly sliced
- small bunch mint, chopped, reserving a few leaves to serve
- small bunch flat-leaf parsley, chopped, reserving a few leaves to serve
- 2 handfuls rocket

Direction

- Boil the barley for 20-25 mins until just tender but with a little bite. Drain.
- Meanwhile, heat oven to 200C/180C fan/gas 6. If using butternut, thickly slice into rounds, flicking out the seeds as you go, or slice small, round squashes into thin wedges. Toss with 1 tbsp oil, the orange zest and seasoning. Spread over a baking sheet and roast for 40 mins until

- golden and tender, turning halfway. Set aside while you finish the dish.
- Mix the orange juice, vinegar and remaining oil with the pearl barley and plenty of seasoning. Stir in the onion and chopped herbs, then layer up on a platter with the squash, rocket and remaining mint and parsley leaves.

Nutrition Information

- Calories: 225 calories
- Total Carbohydrate: 36 grams carbohydrates
- Sugar: 7 grams sugar
- Fiber: 4 grams fiber
- Sodium: 0.03 milligram of sodium
- Total Fat: 6 grams fat
- Saturated Fat: 1 grams saturated fat
- Protein: 5 grams protein

46. Vietnamese Prawn Salad

Serving: 2 | Prep: 20mins | Cook: | Ready in:

Ingredients

- 1 small garlic clove, finely chopped
- 1 small red chilli, deseeded and finely chopped
- 1 tbsp golden caster sugar
- juice 2 limes
- 250g thin rice noodles
- 150g pack cooked tiger prawns, halved along their spine
- ½ cucumber, peeled, deseeded and cut into matchsticks
- 1 carrot, cut into matchsticks or grated
- 6 spring onions, shredded
- handful corianderand/or mint leaves
- 1 tbsp roasted peanuts, chopped

Direction

- To make the dressing, mash the garlic, chilli and sugar using a pestle and mortar. Add the lime juice and 3 tbsp water and stir together. Set aside.
- Get the kettle on, put the noodles into a bowl, then cover with boiling water. Leave to stand for 10 mins until tender, then drain and divide between 2 bowls. 3 Mix the prawns and veg together and divide between the bowls, too. Finish by topping each salad with the herbs and peanuts, then pour over the dressing to serve.

Nutrition Information

- Calories: 579 calories
- Saturated Fat: 3 grams saturated fat
- Total Carbohydrate: 117 grams carbohydrates
- Sugar: 14 grams sugar
- Protein: 27 grams protein
- Sodium: 1.66 milligram of sodium
- Total Fat: 4 grams fat
- Fiber: 2 grams fiber

47. Warm Cauliflower Salad

Serving: 4 | Prep: 15mins | Cook: 35mins | Ready in:

Ingredients

- 1 cauliflower, broken into florets
- 2 tbsp olive oil
- 1 red onion, thinly sliced
- 3 tbsp sherry vinegar
- 1½ tbsp honey
- 3 tbsp raisins
- small bunch dill, snipped
- 3 tbsp toasted, flaked almond
- 50g baby spinach

Direction

- Heat oven to 200C/180C fan/gas 6. Toss the cauliflower with the olive oil, season and roast for 15 mins. Stir in the red onion and carry on roasting for 15-20 mins more until tender.

- While the cauliflower is roasting, mix the vinegar, honey and raisins with some seasoning.
- When the cauliflower is done, stir in the dressing, dill, almonds and spinach, and serve.

Nutrition Information

- Calories: 206 calories
- Total Fat: 11 grams fat
- Sugar: 18 grams sugar
- Fiber: 4 grams fiber
- Sodium: 0.11 milligram of sodium
- Saturated Fat: 1 grams saturated fat
- Total Carbohydrate: 19 grams carbohydrates
- Protein: 8 grams protein

48. Watermelon, Prawn & Avocado Salad

Serving: 4 | Prep: 15mins | Cook: |Ready in:

Ingredients

- 1 small red onion, finely chopped
- 1 fat garlic clove, crushed
- 1 small red chilli, finely chopped
- juice 1 lime
- 1 tbsp rice or white wine vinegar
- 1 tsp caster sugar
- watermelon wedge, deseeded and diced
- 1 avocado, diced
- small bunch coriander leaves, chopped
- 200g cooked tiger prawns, defrosted if frozen

Direction

- Put the onion in a medium bowl with the garlic, chilli, lime juice, vinegar, sugar and some seasoning. Leave to marinate for 10 mins.

- Add the watermelon, avocado, coriander and prawns, then toss gently to serve.

Nutrition Information

- Calories: 179 calories
- Saturated Fat: 1 grams saturated fat
- Protein: 13 grams protein
- Total Carbohydrate: 14 grams carbohydrates
- Total Fat: 8 grams fat
- Fiber: 2 grams fiber
- Sodium: 0.91 milligram of sodium
- Sugar: 13 grams sugar

49. Winter Apple & Squash Panzanella

Serving: 4 | Prep: 20mins | Cook: 40mins |Ready in:

Ingredients

- ½ large butternut squash, cut into chunks
- 4 tbsp extra virgin olive oil
- 6 sage leaves, chopped
- 2 apples, cored and sliced into slim wedges
- 3 tbsp clear honey
- 4 tbsp red wine vinegar
- 200g leftover crusty bread (we used ciabatta), torn into chunks
- 100g hazelnuts, roughly chopped
- 200g bag chopped kale
- 100g dried cranberries

Direction

- Heat oven to 200C/180C fan/gas 6. Put the squash on a baking tray, drizzle with 1 tbsp oil and scatter over the sage and some seasoning. Toss together, then bake for 30 mins.
- Add the apple slices to the tray, drizzle over the honey and toss with the squash. Put the bread on a separate tray and return both trays to the oven. Bake for another 10-15 mins until the squash and apple are tender and starting

to caramelise, and the bread is crisp. Meanwhile, toast the hazelnuts in a small pan until golden. Remove the trays from the oven and set aside to cool a little.

- Whisk the remaining oil, the honey and vinegar in a large bowl with some seasoning. Add the kale, cranberries, hazelnuts, squash apples and toasted bread. Toss everything together, then transfer to a platter or plates to serve.

Nutrition Information

- Calories: 648 calories
- Saturated Fat: 3 grams saturated fat
- Total Carbohydrate: 77 grams carbohydrates
- Fiber: 9 grams fiber
- Sodium: 0.8 milligram of sodium
- Protein: 13 grams protein
- Sugar: 42 grams sugar
- Total Fat: 30 grams fat

Chapter 3: Dairy-Free Dinner Recipes

***

50. Bean & Pepper Chilli

Serving: 4 | Prep: 15mins | Cook: 30mins | Ready in:

Ingredients

- 1 tbsp olive oil
- 1 onion, chopped
- 350g pepper, deseeded and sliced
- 1 tbsp ground cumin
- 1-3 tsp chilli powder, depending on how hot you want your chilli to be
- 1 tbsp sweet smoked paprika

- 400g can kidney bean in chilli sauce
- 400g can mixed bean, drained
- 400g can chopped tomato
- rice, to serve (optional)

Direction

- Heat the oil in a large pan. Add the onion and peppers, and cook for 8 mins until softened. Tip in the spices and cook for 1 min.
- Tip in the beans and tomatoes, bring to the boil and simmer for 15 mins or until the chilli is thickened. Season and serve with rice, if you like.

Nutrition Information

- Calories: 246 calories
- Total Carbohydrate: 29 grams carbohydrates
- Sugar: 14 grams sugar
- Protein: 13 grams protein
- Saturated Fat: 1 grams saturated fat
- Fiber: 15 grams fiber
- Sodium: 0.7 milligram of sodium
- Total Fat: 5 grams fat

51. Chicken Fricassée With New Potatoes & Asparagus

Serving: 6 | Prep: | Cook: 40mins | Ready in:

Ingredients

- 1 tbsp groundnut oil
- 4 lean smoked back bacon rashers, chopped and rind removed
- 6 skinless chicken breast fillets
- 700g new potato, thickly sliced
- 250g asparagus spear, trimmed and diagonally sliced (keep tips whole)
- 225ml dry fruity cider (or ½ a can)
- 1 tbsp cornflour, blended with a little water
- 250ml carton Soya Dream
- 2 tbsp chopped flatleaf parsley

Direction

- Heat the oil in a large frying pan, then fry the bacon for 5 mins on a medium heat until golden. Remove with a slotted spoon and set aside. Add the chicken to the pan, then lightly fry for 4-5 mins to brown on both sides (you may need to brown the chicken in two batches if your pan is not large enough).
- Meanwhile, cook the potatoes in a pan of salted boiling water for 10 mins or until tender. Cook the asparagus in a steamer over the potatoes for 6-8 mins or microwave in a covered dish with 2 tbsp water for 4-5 mins.
- Pour the cider over the chicken, bring to the boil then reduce heat. Put the bacon back in the pan and simmer for 10-15 mins until the chicken is cooked through. Stir in the cornflour paste until lightly thickened, then add the Soya Dream and season. Stir in the drained vegetables and sprinkle with chopped parsley before serving.

Nutrition Information

- Calories: 378 calories
- Total Fat: 13 grams fat
- Saturated Fat: 2 grams saturated fat
- Total Carbohydrate: 24 grams carbohydrates
- Fiber: 2 grams fiber
- Protein: 42 grams protein
- Sodium: 1.11 milligram of sodium

52. Chilli Pepper Pumpkin With Asian Veg

Serving: 2 | Prep: 10mins | Cook: 30mins | Ready in:

Ingredients

- 1 small pumpkin or ½ butternut squash, cut into chunks (seeds removed), no need to peel
- 2 tsp sunflower or vegetable oil
- 1 tsp each mild chilli powder and five spice powder
- 175g thin-stemmed broccoli
- 175g bok choi, quartered
- 2 tbsp low-sodium soy sauce
- 2 tbsp rice wine vinegar
- 1 tbsp honey
- 1 lime, ½ juice, ½ cut into wedges
- few coriander leaves

Direction

- Heat oven to 220C/200C fan/gas 7. Toss the pumpkin in the oil, then sprinkle on the chilli powder, five-spice, 1 tsp black pepper and a pinch of salt, and mix well. Tip into a roasting tray in a single layer and cook for 25-30 mins until tender and starting to caramelise around the edges.
- About 5 mins before the pumpkin is cooked, heat a wok or large frying pan and add the broccoli plus 1-2 tbsp water. Cook for 2-3 mins, then add the bok choi, soy, vinegar and honey, and cook for a further 2-3 mins until the veg is tender. Add the lime juice, then divide between 2 plates with the pumpkin, coriander leaves and lime wedges.

Nutrition Information

- Calories: 248 calories
- Fiber: 7 grams fiber
- Total Fat: 5 grams fat
- Protein: 9 grams protein
- Saturated Fat: 1 grams saturated fat
- Total Carbohydrate: 42 grams carbohydrates
- Sugar: 30 grams sugar
- Sodium: 1.9 milligram of sodium

53. Creamy Tarragon Chicken Bake

Serving: 4 | Prep: 20mins | Cook: 30mins | Ready in:

Ingredients

- 2 tbsp extra-virgin olive oil
- 1 tbsp rice flour (we used Doves Farm)
- 300ml soya milk (we used So Good)
- 4 chicken breasts, skin removed
- 2 red onions, cut into wedges
- 250g punnet cherry tomato, halved
- 250g asparagus spear, blanched
- 1 tsp caster sugar
- 1 tbsp white wine vinegar
- 150ml vegetable stock (we used Kallo yeast-free vegetable stock)
- 3 tbsp chopped tarragon
- 4 tbsp gluten-free breadcrumb (we used Sainsbury's 'Free From' English muffins)
- 1 tbsp grated dairy and lactose-free cheese (we used Cheezly)

Direction

- Mix half the oil and flour in a saucepan (off the heat), then blend in the soya milk (it must be well blended before heating). Bring the sauce slowly to the boil, whisking constantly, then simmer for 1 min. Remove from the heat, cover with greaseproof paper and set aside.
- Heat oven to 200C/fan 180C/gas 6. Heat remaining oil in a frying pan, add the chicken, then fry for 2-3 mins or until brown (it won't be cooked through). Transfer to an ovenproof gratin dish. Add the onions to the pan and fry for 2-3 mins. Spoon over the chicken, then top with the tomatoes and asparagus. Set aside while you prepare the sauce.
- Put the sugar and vinegar into the pan. Stir over medium heat until the sugar is a dark caramel colour, then add the stock. Bring to the boil and simmer for 1 min. Whisk into the milky sauce until blended, season, then add the tarragon. Spoon sauce over the chicken and veg, sprinkle with crumbs and cheese, then bake for 20 mins or until cooked through.

Nutrition Information

- Calories: 320 calories
- Fiber: 3 grams fiber
- Sodium: 0.54 milligram of sodium

- Saturated Fat: 2 grams saturated fat
- Sugar: 8 grams sugar
- Protein: 40 grams protein
- Total Carbohydrate: 18 grams carbohydrates
- Total Fat: 10 grams fat

54. Curry Coconut Fish Parcels

Serving: 2 | Prep: 10mins | Cook: 15mins | Ready in:

Ingredients

- 2 large tilapia fillets, about 125g/4½oz each
- 2 tsp yellow or red curry paste
- 2 tsp desiccated coconut
- zest and juice 1 lime, plus wedges to serve
- 1 tsp soy sauce
- 140g basmati rice
- 2 tbsp sweet chilli sauce
- 1 red chilli, sliced
- 200g cooked thin-stemmed broccoli, to serve

Direction

- Heat oven to 200C/180C fan/gas 6. Tear off 4 large pieces of foil, double them up, then place a fish fillet in the middle of each. Spread over the curry paste. Divide the coconut, lime zest and juice, and soy between each fillet. Bring up the sides of the foil, then scrunch the edges and sides together to make 2 sealed parcels.
- Put the parcels on a baking tray and bake for 10-15 mins. Tip the rice into a pan with plenty of water, and boil for 12-15 mins or until cooked. Drain well. Serve the fish on the rice, drizzle over the chilli sauce and scatter with sliced chilli. Serve with broccoli and lime wedges.

Nutrition Information

- Calories: 438 calories
- Sodium: 1.3 milligram of sodium
- Sugar: 8 grams sugar

- Saturated Fat: 3 grams saturated fat
- Total Carbohydrate: 63 grams carbohydrates
- Total Fat: 6 grams fat
- Fiber: 2 grams fiber
- Protein: 28 grams protein

55. Fisherman's Curry

Serving: 6 | Prep: 20mins | Cook: 25mins | Ready in:

Ingredients

- juice 1 lemon
- 750g boneless, skinless firm white fish, cut into large pieces
- 1 tbsp vegetable oil
- 1 cinnamon stick
- 4 whole cloves
- 4 green cardamom pods
- ½ tsp whole black peppercorns
- 10 fresh curry leaves
- 2 onions, chopped
- 3 green chillies, finely chopped
- 1 tbsp grated ginger
- 4 garlic cloves, finely chopped
- 6 tomatoes, chopped or a 400g can chopped tomatoes
- 1 tsp turmeric
- ½ tsp chilli powder
- 2 tsp ground coriander

Direction

- Stir the lemon juice and 1 tsp salt into the fish pieces and set aside. Heat the oil in a large pan. Add the whole spices and curry leaves, cook for 3-4 mins, then add the onions. Fry until the onions are soft, then add the chillies, ginger and garlic. Tip in the tomatoes and the remaining spices and cook, uncovered, on a low heat for about 5-8 mins. Stir frequently to prevent the spices sticking and burning.
- Pour 150ml water into the pan, bring to a simmer, then add the fish. Cover with a lid and cook for 5 mins more. Serve with rice.

Nutrition Information

- Calories: 152 calories
- Protein: 25 grams protein
- Sodium: 1.1 milligram of sodium
- Total Fat: 3 grams fat
- Total Carbohydrate: 7 grams carbohydrates
- Sugar: 4 grams sugar
- Fiber: 1 grams fiber

56. Florentine Dairy Free Pizza

Serving: 2 | Prep: 25mins | Cook: 20mins | Ready in:

Ingredients

- 2 tbsp olive oil, plus extra for drizzling
- 2 garlic cloves, sliced
- 400g can chopped tomatoes
- 400g frozen spinach, defrosted
- toppings of your choice- anchovies, olives, capers, pepperoni, artichoke hearts, grilled peppers
- 2 eggs
- small handful basil leaves
- 2 handfuls rocket
- juice ½ lemon
- For the base
- 350g strong white flour
- 7g sachet fast-action dried yeast
- 1 tbsp coarse or fine semolina

Direction

- To make the base, tip the flour into the bowl of a table-top mixer (or food processor with a dough attachment). Add 1 tsp salt to one side of the bowl and the yeast to the other. Add 275ml lukewarm water and mix on slow until a sticky dough forms. Turn up the mixer for 5-6 mins until an indent pushed into the dough pops out quickly. Put the dough in a lightly oiled bowl, then cover and leave in a warm place to prove until doubled in size.

- Meanwhile, heat the oil in a frying pan and sizzle the garlic for a few secs, then tip in the tomatoes, season and simmer for 5 mins until the sauce has thickened.
- Heat oven to 220C/200C fan/gas 7. Knead the dough for a few mins, then halve and roll each half as thinly as possible. Lay each base on a baking sheet dusted with the semolina. Divide the tomato sauce between the pizzas, spreading almost to the edge. Dot over the spinach, add your toppings and drizzle with a little oil. Cook for 5 mins, then crack an egg onto each pizza. Swap the baking sheets, then cook for 10 mins more or until bases are cooked through. Drizzle the basil and rocket with a drop of oil and the lemon juice. Scatter over the pizza before eating.

Nutrition Information

- Calories: 827 calories
- Protein: 28 grams protein
- Sodium: 3.4 milligram of sodium
- Total Fat: 17 grams fat
- Saturated Fat: 2 grams saturated fat
- Fiber: 12 grams fiber
- Sugar: 9 grams sugar
- Total Carbohydrate: 140 grams carbohydrates

57. Fruity Caribbean Curry

Serving: 4 | Prep: 10mins | Cook: 50mins | Ready in:

Ingredients

- 2 tsp vegetable or sunflower oil
- 4 chicken drumsticks, skin removed
- 2 large red onions, chopped
- 2 peppers (any colours will do), chopped
- 3-4 tbsp mild curry powder
- 425g can pineapple chunks in unsweetened juice

- 400g can coconut milk
- 400g can kidney beans, drained
- 2-4 tbsp hot pepper sauce (depending on how hot you like it)
- small bunch coriander, chopped
- cooked rice, to serve (we used Tilda coconut rice)

Direction

- Heat the oil in a large frying pan. Add the chicken and brown well on all sides, then transfer to a plate. Add the onions and peppers to the pan, and cook for 5 mins until the veg starts to soften. Return the chicken to the pan and sprinkle in the curry powder, then add the pineapple with its juice, and the coconut milk. Season and simmer, uncovered, for 40 mins until the chicken is tender and the sauce has reduced and thickened a little.
- Add the beans and pepper sauce to the pan. Simmer for another 2-3 mins until the beans are warmed through, then scatter with coriander and serve with cooked rice.

Nutrition Information

- Calories: 458 calories
- Total Fat: 23 grams fat
- Sugar: 23 grams sugar
- Total Carbohydrate: 36 grams carbohydrates
- Sodium: 1.5 milligram of sodium
- Saturated Fat: 16 grams saturated fat
- Protein: 21 grams protein
- Fiber: 11 grams fiber

58. Harissa Lamb & Pepper Kebabs

Serving: 4 | Prep: 15mins | Cook: 10mins | Ready in:

Ingredients

- 2 tbsp harissa paste

- 400g lambsteak, trimmed of any fat and chopped into chunks
- 2 red peppers, chopped into large chunks
- 2 red onions, each cut into 8 wedges through the root so the wedges don't fall apart
- 250g couscous, flavoured or plain
- PLUS 1 tbsp olive oil

Direction

- Heat the grill. In a large bowl, mix the harissa with the oil, then tip in the lamb, peppers and onions. Add some salt and pepper and toss everything together to coat well.
- Thread the lamb, peppers and onions evenly onto 8 skewers and place on a baking tray. Scrape over any leftover marinade.
- Grill for 8-10 mins, turning frequently and basting with any of the juices that run off. Meanwhile, prepare the couscous following pack instructions. Divide the couscous between 4 plates, top with a couple of skewers each and drizzle over any pan juices.

Nutrition Information

- Calories: 351 calories
- Total Carbohydrate: 41 grams carbohydrates
- Protein: 25 grams protein
- Sodium: 0.26 milligram of sodium
- Fiber: 2 grams fiber
- Total Fat: 11 grams fat
- Saturated Fat: 3 grams saturated fat
- Sugar: 8 grams sugar

59. Healthier Chicken Balti

Serving: 4 | Prep: 25mins | Cook: 30mins | Ready in:

Ingredients

- 450g skinless, boneless chicken breast, cut into bite-sized pieces
- 1 tbsp lime juice
- 1 tsp paprika
- ¼ tsp hot chilli powder
- 1½ tbsp sunflower or groundnut oil
- 1 cinnamon stick
- 3 cardamom pods, split
- 1 small to medium green chilli
- ½ tsp cumin seed
- 1 medium onion, coarsely grated
- 2 garlic cloves, very finely chopped
- 2½ cm-piece ginger, grated
- ½ tsp turmeric
- 1 tsp ground cumin
- 1 tsp ground coriander
- 1 tsp garam masala
- 250ml organic passata
- 1 red pepper, deseeded, cut into small chunks
- 1 medium tomato, chopped
- 85g baby spinach leaves
- handful fresh coriander, chopped
- chapatis or basmati rice, to serve (optional)

Direction

- Put the chicken in a medium bowl. Mix in the lime juice, paprika, chilli powder and a grinding of black pepper (step 1), then leave to marinate for at least 15 mins, preferably a bit longer.
- Heat 1 tbsp of the oil in a large non-stick wok or sauté pan. Tip in the cinnamon stick, cardamom pods, whole chilli and cumin seeds, and stir-fry briefly just to colour and release their fragrance (step 2). Stir in the onion, garlic and ginger and fry over a medium-high heat for 3-4 mins until the onion starts to turn brown. Add the remaining oil, then drop in the chicken and stir-fry for 2-3 mins or until it no longer looks raw. Mix the turmeric, cumin, ground coriander and garam masala together. Tip into the pan, lower the heat to medium and cook for 2 mins (step 3). Pour in the passata and 150ml water, then drop in the chunks of pepper. When starting to bubble, lower the heat and simmer for 15-20 mins or until the chicken is tender.
- Stir in the tomato, simmer for 2-3 mins, then add the spinach and turn it over in the pan to

just wilt. Season with a little salt. If you want to thin down the sauce, splash in a little more water. Remove the cinnamon stick, chilli and cardamom pods, if you wish, before serving. Scatter with fresh coriander and serve with warm chapatis or basmati rice, if you like.

Nutrition Information

- Calories: 217 calories
- Fiber: 2.5 grams fiber
- Sodium: 0.5 milligram of sodium
- Total Fat: 6.6 grams fat
- Total Carbohydrate: 10.2 grams carbohydrates
- Sugar: 8.2 grams sugar
- Protein: 30.2 grams protein
- Saturated Fat: 1.3 grams saturated fat

60. Herby Pork With Apple & Chicory Salad

Serving: 4 | Prep: 10mins | Cook: 25mins | Ready in:

Ingredients

- 400g pork tenderloin, trimmed of any fat and sinew
- 1tbsp walnut oil
- 2tsp wholegrain mustard
- 1tbsp each chopped tarragon and parsley
- juice 1 lemon
- 1tbsp honey
- 2 large eating apples, cored and sliced
- 270g pack chicory, leaves separated

Direction

- Heat oven to 200C/180C fan/gas 6. Rub the pork with 1 tsp oil, 1 tsp mustard and some seasoning. Brown, transfer to a baking tray and press on half the herbs. Roast for 15 mins until just cooked.
- To make the salad, mix the lemon juice, honey and remaining walnut oil and mustard

together. Season and toss through the apples, chicory and remaining herbs. Serve the pork sliced, with the salad on the side.

Nutrition Information

- Calories: 215 calories
- Sodium: 0.3 milligram of sodium
- Total Fat: 8 grams fat
- Total Carbohydrate: 15 grams carbohydrates
- Saturated Fat: 2 grams saturated fat
- Protein: 23 grams protein
- Sugar: 14 grams sugar
- Fiber: 2 grams fiber

61. Honey & Orange Roast Sea Bass With Lentils

Serving: 2 | Prep: 15mins | Cook: 10mins | Ready in:

Ingredients

- 2 large skin-on sea bass fillets (or other white fish - see tip)
- zest and juice ½ orange
- 2 tsp clear honey
- 2 tsp wholegrain mustard
- 2 tbsp olive oil
- 250g pouch ready-to-eat puy lentils
- 100g watercress
- small bunch parsley, chopped
- small bunch dill, chopped

Direction

- Heat oven to 200C/180C fan/gas 6. Place each sea bass fillet, skin-side down, on individual squares of foil. Mix together the orange zest, honey, mustard, 1 tbsp olive oil and some seasoning, and drizzle it over the fillets. Pull the sides of the foil up and twist the edges together to make individual parcels. Place the parcels on a baking tray and bake in the oven for 10 mins until the fish is just cooked and flakes easily when pressed with a knife.

- Warm the lentils following pack instructions, then mix with the orange juice, remaining oil, the watercress, herbs and seasoning. Divide the lentils between 2 plates and top each with a sea bass fillet. Drizzle over any roasting juices that are caught in the foil and serve immediately.

Nutrition Information

- Calories: 495 calories
- Protein: 44 grams protein
- Sodium: 1.9 milligram of sodium
- Saturated Fat: 3 grams saturated fat
- Total Carbohydrate: 33 grams carbohydrates
- Sugar: 9 grams sugar
- Total Fat: 18 grams fat
- Fiber: 12 grams fiber

62. Jerk Pork & Pineapple Skewers With Black Beans & Rice

Serving: 4 | Prep: 10mins | Cook: 10mins | Ready in:

Ingredients

- 400g pork fillet, cut into 4cm chunks
- 2 tbsp jerk or Creole seasoning
- 1 tsp ground allspice
- 1 tbsp hot chilli sauce, plus extra to serve (optional)
- 3 limes, zest and juice 1, other 2 cut into wedges to serve
- ½ small pineapple, peeled, cored and cut into 4cm chunks
- 1 tbsp vegetable oil
- 200g basmati rice
- 400g can black bean, drained and rinsed

Direction

- Mix together the pork, jerk seasoning, allspice, chilli sauce, if using, lime zest and juice, and some seasoning. Thread the pork and pineapple onto metal skewers (or pre-soaked wooden skewers) and brush with the oil.
- Cook rice following pack instructions. Drain well, then put back in the saucepan with the beans, stir and keep warm.
- Meanwhile, heat a griddle pan until very hot. Cook the skewers for 3 mins on each side until nicely charred and the pork is cooked through. Serve skewers with the beans and rice, extra chilli sauce, if you like, and lime wedges for squeezing over.

Nutrition Information

- Calories: 451 calories
- Total Fat: 10 grams fat
- Total Carbohydrate: 57 grams carbohydrates
- Sodium: 0.2 milligram of sodium
- Sugar: 7 grams sugar
- Protein: 30 grams protein
- Saturated Fat: 3 grams saturated fat
- Fiber: 6 grams fiber

63. Lemon Spaghetti With Tuna & Broccoli

Serving: 4 | Prep: 5mins | Cook: 10mins | Ready in:

Ingredients

- 350g spaghetti
- 250g broccoli, cut into small florets
- 2 shallots, finely chopped
- 85g pitted green olive, halved
- 2 tbsp caper, drained
- 198g can tuna in oil
- zest and juice 1 lemon
- 1 tbsp olive oil, plus extra for drizzling

Direction

- Boil the spaghetti in salted water for 6 mins. Add the broccoli and boil for 4 mins more or until both are just tender.
- Meanwhile, mix the shallots, olives, capers, tuna and lemon zest and juice in a roomy serving bowl. Drain the pasta and broccoli, add to the bowl and toss really well with the olive oil and lots of black pepper. Serve with a little extra olive oil drizzled over.

Nutrition Information

- Calories: 440 calories
- Saturated Fat: 2 grams saturated fat
- Sodium: 1.4 milligram of sodium
- Total Fat: 11 grams fat
- Sugar: 4 grams sugar
- Total Carbohydrate: 62 grams carbohydrates
- Fiber: 5 grams fiber
- Protein: 23 grams protein

64. Mexican Chicken Stew

Serving: 4 | Prep: 20mins | Cook: 25mins | Ready in:

Ingredients

- 1 tbsp vegetable oil
- 1 medium onion, finely chopped
- 3 garlic cloves, finely chopped
- ½ tsp dark brown sugar
- 1 tsp chipotle paste (we used Discovery)
- 400g can chopped tomatoes
- 4 skinless, boneless chicken breasts
- 1 small red onion, sliced into rings
- a few coriander leaves
- corn tortillas, or rice to serve

Direction

- Heat the oil in a medium saucepan. Add the onion and cook for 5 mins or until softened and starting to turn golden, adding the garlic for the final min. Stir in the sugar, chipotle

paste and tomatoes. Put the chicken into the pan, spoon over the sauce, and simmer gently for 20 mins until the chicken has cooked (add a splash of water if the sauce gets too dry).
- Remove the chicken from the pan and shred with 2 forks, then stir back into the sauce. Scatter with a little red onion, the coriander, and serve with remaining red onion, tortillas or rice.
- If you want to use a slow cooker, cook the onion and garlic as above, then put into your slow cooker with the sugar, chipotle, tomatoes and chicken. Cover and cook on High for 2 hours. Remove the chicken and shred then serve as above.

Nutrition Information

- Calories: 203 calories
- Saturated Fat: 1 grams saturated fat
- Protein: 35 grams protein
- Total Fat: 5 grams fat
- Sugar: 4 grams sugar
- Sodium: 0.37 milligram of sodium
- Fiber: 2 grams fiber
- Total Carbohydrate: 6 grams carbohydrates

65. Pot Roast Loin Of Pork In Cider With Celeriac

Serving: 6 | Prep: 20mins | Cook: 1hours45mins | Ready in:

Ingredients

- 2 ½kg pork loin, bone in
- 1 tbsp olive oil
- 100g smoked bacon lardons
- 300g banana shallots, halved horizontally
- 500-600g celeriac, peeled and cut into 3cm chunks
- 6 thyme sprigs
- 1 garlic bulb, halved
- 600ml dry cider

- 140g frozen peas
- mash, to serve

Direction

- Heat oven to 180C/160C fan/gas 4. Season the pork and put in a large roasting tin.
- Heat a large frying pan, add the oil and fry the lardons, shallots, celeriac and thyme until golden brown. Arrange around the pork with the garlic bulb.
- Add the cider to the frying pan, bring to the boil, then pour around the pork. Cover with foil and roast for 1 hr. Remove the foil and cook, uncovered, for a further 45 mins.
- Finally, add the peas and cook for 3 mins more. Leave the pork to stand, covered, for 15 mins before carving. Serve with buttery mash (add the soft roasted garlic cloves if you like) to soak up the delicious juices.

Nutrition Information

- Calories: 575 calories
- Total Fat: 33 grams fat
- Saturated Fat: 11 grams saturated fat
- Total Carbohydrate: 9 grams carbohydrates
- Protein: 50 grams protein
- Sugar: 6 grams sugar
- Fiber: 7 grams fiber
- Sodium: 0.9 milligram of sodium

66. Pumpkin Curry With Chickpeas

Serving: 4 | Prep: 20mins | Cook: 20mins | Ready in:

Ingredients

- 1 tbsp sunflower oil
- 3 tbsp Thai yellow curry paste, or vegetarian alternative
- 2 onions, finely chopped
- 3 large stalks lemongrass, bashed with the back of a knife

- 6 cardamom pods
- 1 tbsp mustard seed
- 1 piece pumpkin or a small squash (about 1kg)
- 250ml vegetable stock
- 400ml can reduced-fat coconut milk
- 400g can chickpea, drained and rinsed
- 2 limes
- large handful mint leaves
- naan bread, to serve

Direction

- Heat the oil in a sauté pan, then gently fry the curry paste with the onions, lemongrass, cardamom and mustard seed for 2-3 mins until fragrant. Stir the pumpkin or squash into the pan and coat in the paste, then pour in the stock and coconut milk. Bring everything to a simmer, add the chickpeas, then cook for about 10 mins until the pumpkin is tender. The curry can now be cooled and frozen for up to 1 month.
- Squeeze the juice of one lime into the curry, then cut the other lime into wedges to serve alongside. Just before serving, tear over mint leaves, then bring to the table with the lime wedges and warm naan breads.

Nutrition Information

- Calories: 293 calories
- Total Fat: 18 grams fat
- Saturated Fat: 10 grams saturated fat
- Total Carbohydrate: 26 grams carbohydrates
- Sugar: 10 grams sugar
- Protein: 9 grams protein
- Sodium: 1.32 milligram of sodium

67. Quinoa Stew With Squash, Prunes & Pomegranate

Serving: 4 | Prep: 15mins | Cook: 40mins | Ready in:

Ingredients

- 1 small butternut squash, deseeded and cubed
- 2 tbsp olive oil
- 1 large onion, thinly sliced
- 1 garlic clove, chopped
- 1 tbsp finely chopped ginger
- 1 tsp ras-el-hanout or Middle Eastern spice mix
- 200g quinoa
- 5 prunes, roughly chopped
- juice 1 lemon
- 600ml vegetable stock
- seeds from 1 pomegranate
- small handful mint leaves

Direction

- Heat oven to 200C/180C fan/gas 6. Put the squash on a baking tray and toss with 1 tbsp of the oil. Season well and roast for 30-35 mins or until soft.
- Meanwhile, heat the remaining oil in a big saucepan. Add the onion, garlic and ginger, season and cook for 10 mins. Add the spice and quinoa, and cook for another couple of mins. Add the prunes, lemon juice and stock, bring to the boil, then cover and simmer for 25 mins.
- When everything is tender, stir the squash through the stew. Spoon into bowls and scatter with pomegranate seeds and mint to serve.

Nutrition Information

- Calories: 318 calories
- Fiber: 6 grams fiber
- Sugar: 20 grams sugar
- Total Carbohydrate: 50 grams carbohydrates
- Protein: 11 grams protein
- Sodium: 0.5 milligram of sodium
- Saturated Fat: 1 grams saturated fat
- Total Fat: 9 grams fat

68. Rosemary Chicken With Oven Roasted Ratatouille

Serving: 4 | Prep: 15mins | Cook: 40mins | Ready in:

Ingredients

- 1 aubergine, cut into chunky pieces
- 2 courgettes, sliced into half-moons
- 3 mixed peppers, deseeded and roughly chopped
- 2 tsp finely chopped rosemary, plus 4 small sprigs
- 2 large garlic cloves, crushed
- 3 tbsp olive oil
- 4 skinless, boneless chicken breasts
- 250g cherry or baby plum tomato, halved

Direction

- Heat oven to 200C/180C fan/gas 6. In a large roasting tin, toss together the aubergine, courgettes and peppers with half the chopped rosemary, half the garlic, 2 tbsp oil and some seasoning. Spread out the vegetables in an even layer, then roast in the oven for 20 mins.
- Meanwhile, mix remaining rosemary, garlic and oil together. Slash each of the chicken breasts 4-5 times with a sharp knife, brush over the flavoured oil, season and chill for 15 mins.
- After veg have cooked for 20 mins, stir in the tomatoes. Make spaces in the roasting tin and nestle the chicken breasts amongst the vegetables. Place a rosemary sprig on top of each chicken breast. Return the tin to the oven for 18-20 mins, until the chicken is cooked through and the vegetables are lightly caramelised. Serve with some new potatoes, if you like.

Nutrition Information

- Calories: 288 calories
- Protein: 37 grams protein
- Saturated Fat: 2 grams saturated fat
- Total Carbohydrate: 11 grams carbohydrates

- Fiber: 5 grams fiber
- Sodium: 0.25 milligram of sodium
- Total Fat: 11 grams fat
- Sugar: 10 grams sugar

69. Sea Bass & Seafood Italian One Pot

Serving: 4 | Prep: 15mins | Cook: 45mins | Ready in:

Ingredients

- 2 tbsp olive oil
- 1 fennel bulb, halved and sliced, fronds kept separate to garnish
- 2 garlic cloves, sliced
- ½ red chilli, chopped
- 250g cleaned squid, sliced into rings
- bunch basil, leaves and stalks separated, stalks tied together, leaves roughly chopped
- 400g can chopped tomato
- 150ml white wine
- 2 large handfuls of mussels or clams
- 8 large raw prawns (whole look nicest)
- 4 sea bass fillets (about 140g/5oz each)
- crusty bread, to serve

Direction

- Heat the oil in a large saucepan with a tight-fitting lid, then add the fennel, garlic and chilli. Fry until softened, then add the squid, basil stalks, tomatoes and wine. Simmer over a low heat for 35 mins until the squid is tender and the sauce has thickened slightly, then season.
- Scatter the mussels and prawns over the sauce, lay the sea bass fillets on top, cover, turn up the heat and cook hard for 5 mins. Serve scattered with the basil leaves and fennel fronds, with crusty bread.

Nutrition Information

- Calories: 329 calories
- Saturated Fat: 2 grams saturated fat
- Fiber: 2 grams fiber
- Sodium: 1 milligram of sodium
- Total Carbohydrate: 7 grams carbohydrates
- Protein: 45 grams protein
- Sugar: 4 grams sugar
- Total Fat: 11 grams fat

70. Simmered Squid

Serving: Serves 4 as a main, 6 as a starter | Prep: 20mins | Cook: 1hours15mins | Ready in:

Ingredients

- 1 tbsp olive oil, plus extra for drizzling
- 1kg prepared squid and tentacles, cleaned and cut into thick rings
- 2 onions, chopped
- 3 garlic cloves, sliced
- pinch of chilli flakes
- 1 tsp fennel seed
- 3 bay leaves
- 1 tbsp rosemary, roughly chopped
- pinch of sugar
- 3 tbsp red wine vinegar
- 400g can chopped tomato
- large glass of red wine (about 200ml)
- To serve
- handful chopped coriander
- zest ½ orange

Direction

- Heat the olive oil in a shallow saucepan or flameproof casserole and add the squid, onions and garlic. Add the dry ingredients and simmer until all the liquid has evaporated and the onions are tender, about 15 mins. Add the vinegar and chopped tomatoes, simmer for 1 min, then pour over the red wine and season. Simmer very gently on the lowest heat, stirring occasionally, for 1 hr or until the sauce is rich and the squid is really tender.

- Turn off the heat, leave to cool slightly, then drizzle with a little more olive oil and scatter with the coriander and orange zest.

Nutrition Information

- Calories: 352 calories
- Total Fat: 8 grams fat
- Saturated Fat: 2 grams saturated fat
- Total Carbohydrate: 12 grams carbohydrates
- Sugar: 7 grams sugar
- Fiber: 2 grams fiber
- Protein: 41 grams protein
- Sodium: 0.8 milligram of sodium

71. Singapore Noodles

Serving: 4 | Prep: 15mins | Cook: 30mins | Ready in:

Ingredients

- 3 tbsp teriyaki sauce
- ½ tsp Chinese five-spice powder
- 2 tsp medium Madras curry powder
- 300g/11oz pork tenderloin, trimmed of any fat
- 140g medium egg noodle
- 1 tbsp sunflower oil
- 2 x 300g packs fresh mixed stir-fry vegetables
- 100g cooked prawn, thawed if frozen

Direction

- Mix the teriyaki sauce, five-spice and curry powders. Add half to the pork, turning to coat, and leave to marinate for 15 mins.
- Heat oven to 200C/180C fan/ gas 6. Remove pork from the marinade and put on a small baking tray lined with foil. Roast for 15-20 mins.
- Meanwhile, cook the noodles following pack instructions, but reduce the cooking time by 1 min. Refresh in cold water and drain very well.

- Transfer the pork to a chopping board and rest for 5 mins. Set a large non-stick frying pan or wok over a medium-high heat. Add the oil and stir-fry the veg for 3-4 mins. Cut the pork in half lengthways, then thinly slice. Tip into the pan, with the prawns, noodles and remaining marinade. Toss together for 2-3 mins until hot.

Nutrition Information

- Calories: 293 calories
- Total Carbohydrate: 32 grams carbohydrates
- Sodium: 1.7 milligram of sodium
- Total Fat: 6 grams fat
- Saturated Fat: 1 grams saturated fat
- Protein: 27 grams protein
- Fiber: 4 grams fiber
- Sugar: 7 grams sugar

72. Soba Noodle & Edamame Salad With Grilled Tofu

Serving: 4 | Prep: 15mins | Cook: 15mins | Ready in:

Ingredients

- 140g soba noodles
- 300g fresh or frozen podded edamame (soy) beans
- 4 spring onions, shredded
- 300g bag beansprouts
- 1 cucumber, peeled, halved lengthways, deseeded with a teaspoon and sliced
- 250g block firm tofu, patted dry and thickly sliced
- 1 tsp oil
- handful coriander leaves, to serve
- For the dressing
- 3 tbsp mirin
- 2 tsp tamari
- 2 tbsp orange juice
- 1 red chilli, deseeded, if you like, and finely chopped

Direction

- Heat dressing ingredients in your smallest saucepan, simmer for 30 secs, then set aside.
- Boil noodles following the pack instructions, adding the edamame beans for the final 2 mins cooking time. Rinse under very cold water, drain thoroughly and tip into a large bowl with the spring onions, beansprouts, cucumber, sesame oil and warm dressing. Season if you like.
- Brush tofu with the veg oil, season and griddle or grill for 2-3 mins each side – the tofu is very delicate so turn carefully. Top the salad with the tofu, scatter with coriander and serve

Nutrition Information

- Calories: 331 calories
- Total Carbohydrate: 48 grams carbohydrates
- Sugar: 7 grams sugar
- Total Fat: 7 grams fat
- Protein: 21 grams protein
- Sodium: 1.24 milligram of sodium
- Fiber: 5 grams fiber
- Saturated Fat: 1 grams saturated fat

73. Spanish Seafood Rice

Serving: 4 | Prep: 10mins | Cook: 35mins | Ready in:

Ingredients

- 1 tbsp olive oil
- 1 onion, finely chopped
- 1 red and 1 yellow pepper, deseeded and sliced
- 2 garlic cloves, sliced
- 250g paella rice
- 850ml hot vegetable stock(we used Kallo very low salt stock)
- pinch saffron
- 400g seafood mix(we used a bag of frozen mixed seafood, defrosted before use)

- juice ½ small lemon
- small handful flat-leaf parsley, roughly chopped

Direction

- Heat the oil in a large saucepan and soften the onion for 6-7 mins. Add the pepper and garlic, cook for 2 mins more, then stir in the paella rice and cook for 1 min, stirring to coat.
- Pour in the stock, add the saffron and bring to the boil. Cook, uncovered, at a gentle bubble, for 20 mins, stirring occasionally until the rice is tender.
- Stir in the seafood and lemon juice and cook for 2 mins or until piping hot and completely cooked through. Serve in warm bowls scattered with the parsley.

Nutrition Information

- Calories: 369 calories
- Protein: 23 grams protein
- Total Carbohydrate: 58 grams carbohydrates
- Fiber: 7 grams fiber
- Saturated Fat: 1 grams saturated fat
- Sugar: 6 grams sugar
- Sodium: 1.05 milligram of sodium
- Total Fat: 7 grams fat

74. Spicy Seafood Stew With Tomatoes & Lime

Serving: 6 | Prep: 15mins | Cook: 30mins | Ready in:

Ingredients

- 2 dried ancho or guajillo chillies
- 1 tbsp olive oil
- 1 large onion, chopped
- 4 garlic cloves, chopped
- 1 tsp chipotle paste or 1 tsp smoked hot paprika (pimentón)
- 1 tsp ground cumin

- 700ml chicken stock
- 250g chopped tomato, from a can
- 200g large peeled raw prawn
- 300g halibut or other firm white fish fillets, cut into 2.5cm pieces
- 300g clam
- 500g small new potato, halved and boiled
- juice 2 limes
- To serve
- lime wedges
- 1 avocado, chopped
- handful coriander leaves
- 1 small red onion, finely diced
- corn tortillas, sliced and baked

Direction

- Toast the chillies in a hot dry frying pan for a few moments (they will puff up a bit), then remove. Deseed and stem chillies, and soak in boiling water for 15 mins.
- Heat the olive oil in a large saucepan over a medium heat. Add the onion and garlic, season and cook for about 5 mins or until softened. Add the chipotle paste, reconstituted chillies, cumin, stock and tomatoes. Sauté for 5 mins, then purée until very fine in a blender. Pour back into the pan and bring to the boil. Reduce the heat and simmer for 10 mins. When close to eating, add the prawns, fish fillets, clams and potatoes. Place a lid on top and cook for 5 mins over a medium-high heat. Add the lime juice and serve with lime wedges, avocado, coriander, red onion and tortilla chips for sprinkling over.

Nutrition Information

- Calories: 347 calories
- Total Carbohydrate: 28 grams carbohydrates
- Protein: 44 grams protein
- Saturated Fat: 1 grams saturated fat
- Total Fat: 6 grams fat
- Sugar: 7 grams sugar
- Sodium: 1.1 milligram of sodium
- Fiber: 4 grams fiber

75. Spinach & Chickpea Curry

Serving: 4 | Prep: 5mins | Cook: 15mins | Ready in:

Ingredients

- 2 tbsp mild curry paste
- 1 onion, chopped
- 400g can cherry tomatoes
- 2 x 400g cans chickpeas, drained and rinsed
- 250g bag baby leaf spinach
- squeeze lemon juice
- basmati rice, to serve

Direction

- Heat the curry paste in a large non-stick frying pan. Once it starts to split, add the onion and cook for 2 mins to soften. Tip in the tomatoes and bubble for 5 mins or until the sauce has reduced.
- Add the chickpeas and some seasoning, then cook for 1 min more. Take off the heat, then tip in the spinach and allow the heat of the pan to wilt the leaves. Season, add the lemon juice, and serve with basmati rice.

Nutrition Information

- Calories: 203 calories
- Total Carbohydrate: 28 grams carbohydrates
- Sugar: 5 grams sugar
- Fiber: 6 grams fiber
- Protein: 9 grams protein
- Sodium: 1.5 milligram of sodium
- Total Fat: 4 grams fat

76. Super Veg Pasta

Serving: 6 | Prep: 15mins | Cook: 30mins | Ready in:

Ingredients

- 2 red peppers, quartered and deseeded
- 2 tbsp olive oil
- 1 fennel bulb, roughly chopped
- 1 onion, roughly chopped
- 1 large carrot, roughly chopped
- 2 garlic cloves, crushed
- ¼ tsp crushed chillies
- 1 tsp fennel seeds
- 2 tbsp tomato purée
- 400g can chopped tomatoes
- 600ml vegetable stock
- 1 tsp caster sugar
- small handful basil, leaves shredded
- 500g bag fresh egg pasta, cooked

Direction

- Heat the grill and pop the peppers, skin-side up, underneath for 10 mins or until beginning to char. Transfer to a bowl, cover and set aside. When cool enough to handle, peel off the skin and cut the flesh into strips.
- Heat the oil in a large saucepan and cook the fennel, onion and carrot for 8-10 mins until softened. Stir in the garlic, crushed chillies, fennel seeds and tomato purée, cook for 2 mins, then add the canned tomatoes, stock and sugar. Simmer, uncovered, for 15 mins or until the vegetables are completely soft.
- Take out a couple of spoonfuls of the sauce (this will later add texture), then blend the rest in the saucepan until almost smooth with a stick blender. Simmer for 5 mins to thicken, then stir in the reserved sauce, shredded basil and peppers. Serve with the pasta.

Nutrition Information

- Calories: 323 calories
- Sugar: 11 grams sugar
- Fiber: 6 grams fiber
- Total Carbohydrate: 58 grams carbohydrates
- Sodium: 0.45 milligram of sodium
- Total Fat: 6 grams fat
- Protein: 12 grams protein

- Saturated Fat: 1 grams saturated fat

77. Veggie Thai Red Curry

Serving: 4 | Prep: 30mins | Cook: 20mins | Ready in:

Ingredients

- 200g firm tofu, cubed
- 4-5 tbsp soy sauce
- juice 3 limes
- 2 red chillies, 1 finely chopped, 1 sliced into rounds
- 2 tbsp vegetable oil
- 400ml can reduced-fat coconut milk
- 1 courgette, chopped into chunks
- 1 small aubergine, chopped into chunks
- ½ red pepper, deseeded and chopped into chunks
- 140g mushrooms, halved
- 140g sugar snap pea
- 20g pack basil, leaves picked
- 1 tsp brown sugar
- jasmine rice, to serve
- For the paste
- 3 red chillies
- 1 lemongrass, roughly chopped
- 3 shallots, roughly chopped
- ½ red pepper, deseeded and roughly chopped
- zest 1 lime
- stalks from 20g pack coriander
- thumb-size piece ginger, grated
- 2 garlic cloves
- 1 tsp freshly ground pepper
- 1 tsp ground coriander

Direction

- Whizz the paste ingredients in a food processor. Marinate the tofu in 2 tbsp soy sauce, juice 1 lime and the chopped chilli.
- Heat half the oil in a large pan. Add 3-4 tbsp paste and fry for 2 mins. Stir in the coconut milk with 100ml water, the courgette,

aubergine and pepper and cook for 10 mins until almost tender.

- Drain the tofu, pat dry, then fry in the remaining oil in a small pan until golden.
- Add the mushrooms, sugar snaps and most of the basil to the curry, then season with the sugar, remaining lime juice and soy sauce. Cook for 4 mins until the mushrooms are tender, then add the tofu and heat through. Scatter with sliced chilli and basil and serve with jasmine rice.

Nutrition Information

- Calories: 233 calories
- Sodium: 3.06 milligram of sodium
- Saturated Fat: 10 grams saturated fat
- Total Fat: 18 grams fat
- Total Carbohydrate: 11 grams carbohydrates
- Sugar: 7 grams sugar
- Fiber: 3 grams fiber
- Protein: 8 grams protein

78. Zesty Lamb Chops With Crushed Kidney Beans

Serving: 4 | Prep: 15mins | Cook: 20mins | Ready in:

Ingredients

- 8 lamb chops
- 2 tbsp olive oil
- juice and zest 1 lemon
- 1-2 red chillies, deseeded and finely chopped
- 1 garlic clove, crushed
- 2 x 400g cans red kidney beans, drained
- small pack mint, leaves picked and finely chopped
- mixed green leaves such as rocket and watercress, to serve

Direction

- Heat a griddle pan over a high heat. Brush the lamb chops with 1 tbsp oil, then rub all over with the lemon zest and some seasoning. Griddle for 3-4 mins each side for slightly pink meat, or a little longer for well done. You may need to do this in 2 batches. Remove from the pan, wrap in foil and leave to rest for 10 mins.
- Gently fry the remaining oil, the chillies and garlic in a saucepan for 2-3 mins. Add the kidney beans and gently crush them with a potato masher, then continue to cook for 3 mins until the beans are warm. Stir in the lemon juice, mint and seasoning, and serve with the chops and mixed leaves.

Nutrition Information

- Calories: 519 calories
- Total Fat: 24 grams fat
- Total Carbohydrate: 21 grams carbohydrates
- Sugar: 4 grams sugar
- Sodium: 1.5 milligram of sodium
- Saturated Fat: 8 grams saturated fat
- Fiber: 10 grams fiber
- Protein: 50 grams protein

Chapter 4: Dairy-Free Snack Recipes

***

79. Apple Crisps

Serving: Makes roughly 16 | Prep: 5mins | Cook: 40mins | Ready in:

Ingredients

- 1 apple

Direction

- Heat oven to 140C/120C fan/gas 1. Thinly slice the apple through the core – use a mandolin, if you have one, to get thin slices. Arrange the slices on a baking tray lined with parchment and bake for 40 mins. Cool until crisp.

Nutrition Information

- Calories: 5 calories
- Total Carbohydrate: 1 grams carbohydrates
- Sugar: 1 grams sugar
- Sodium: 0.1 milligram of sodium

80. Baked Skinny Fries

Serving: 4 | Prep: 10mins | Cook: 40mins | Ready in:

Ingredients

- 1 tbsp vegetable oil
- 2 tsp fine cornmeal or polenta
- ½ tsp paprika
- ¼ tsp garlic powder
- 2 large potatoes, cut into 1cm-thick chips

Direction

- Heat oven to 200C/180C fan/gas 6. Pour the oil onto a baking tray and put in the oven for 3 mins. Mix the cornmeal or polenta, paprika and garlic powder together and season. Toss the chips in the mix, then tip onto the tray. Shake well, then cook for 40 mins, shaking halfway through, until crisp and golden.

Nutrition Information

- Calories: 118 calories
- Sugar: 1 grams sugar
- Fiber: 2 grams fiber
- Protein: 3 grams protein

- Total Fat: 3 grams fat
- Total Carbohydrate: 20 grams carbohydrates

81. Beetroot & Apple Salad Pots

Serving: 8 | Prep: 15mins | Cook: | Ready in:

Ingredients

- 250g cooked beetroot, diced into 1cm cubes
- 2 apples, diced into 1cm cubes
- 2 celery sticks, finely sliced
- 50g walnut, roughly chopped
- handful parsley, chopped
- 3 tbsp walnut oil
- 1 tbsp red wine vinegar

Direction

- Put the beetroot, apples, celery, walnuts and parsley in a bowl. Whisk together the walnut oil, vinegar and some seasoning, pour over the beetroot salad and mix well. Divide between small glasses or teacups and chill until ready to serve. Can be made up to 3 hrs ahead.

Nutrition Information

- Calories: 143 calories
- Fiber: 2 grams fiber
- Protein: 2 grams protein
- Sodium: 0.1 milligram of sodium
- Total Fat: 11 grams fat
- Sugar: 8 grams sugar
- Saturated Fat: 1 grams saturated fat
- Total Carbohydrate: 8 grams carbohydrates

82. Bombay Popcorn Mix

Serving: 4 | Prep: 5mins | Cook: 25mins | Ready in:

Ingredients

- 400g can chickpea, drained and dried
- 1 tsp vegetable oil
- 50g butter
- 2 tsp garam masala
- 1 tsp curry powder
- 70g bag salted popcorn
- 85g peanut
- 100g sultana

Direction

- Heat oven to 200C/180C fan/gas 6. Tip the chickpeas onto a baking tray with the oil. Season, shake well to coat, then bake for 25 mins.
- Meanwhile, melt the butter in a microwave. Mix in the garam masala, curry power and some salt and pepper. Tip the popcorn, peanuts and sultanas into a bowl, add the baked chickpeas and pour over the spiced butter. Stir everything well to coat.

Nutrition Information

- Calories: 458 calories
- Total Fat: 27 grams fat
- Sugar: 18 grams sugar
- Fiber: 5 grams fiber
- Protein: 11 grams protein
- Sodium: 1 milligram of sodium
- Saturated Fat: 9 grams saturated fat
- Total Carbohydrate: 39 grams carbohydrates

83. Butternut & Harissa Hummus

Serving: 6 | Prep: 10mins | Cook: 45mins | Ready in:

Ingredients

- ½ butternut squash (about 400g), peeled and cut into 2cm pieces
- 3 garlic cloves, unpeeled
- 2 tbsp olive oil
- 3 tbsp tahini paste

- 1 tbsp harissa, plus a little extra for drizzling
- 400g can chickpeas, drained and rinsed

Direction

- Heat oven to 200C/180C fan/gas 6. Put the butternut squash and garlic cloves in a roasting tin, season well and add 100ml water. Cover the tin with foil and bake for 45 mins, until the squash is really tender. Leave to cool.
- Tip the squash into a food processor with any juices from the tin. Add the garlic cloves, squeezed out of their skins. Add the remaining ingredients, season with salt and blend to a paste.
- Scrape the hummus into a bowl. Drizzle with extra harissa before serving.

Nutrition Information

- Calories: 155 calories
- Protein: 4 grams protein
- Total Fat: 9 grams fat
- Saturated Fat: 1 grams saturated fat
- Sodium: 0.4 milligram of sodium
- Fiber: 3 grams fiber
- Total Carbohydrate: 13 grams carbohydrates
- Sugar: 3 grams sugar

84. Chargrilled Veg Hummus With Dippers

Serving: 4 | Prep: 10mins | Cook: | Ready in:

Ingredients

- 350g frozen chargrilled vegetables, defrosted
- 400g can chickpeas, drained
- 1 garlic clove, chopped
- juice ½ lemon
- 1 tsp olive oil
- 2 wholemeal pitta breads, toasted and sliced
- 100g radishes, scrubbed
- 2 carrots, cut into batons

- 3 celery sticks, cut into batons

Direction

- Tip the vegetables, most of the chickpeas, garlic and lemon juice into the bowl of a food processor with some seasoning, then whizz until smooth.
- Put the hummus into a serving bowl. Scatter over the reserved chickpeas and the olive oil. Serve with toasted pitta slices and the vegetables to dip in.

Nutrition Information

- Calories: 266 calories
- Sugar: 8.6 grams sugar
- Protein: 12 grams protein
- Total Fat: 5.9 grams fat
- Sodium: 0.4 milligram of sodium
- Fiber: 9.1 grams fiber
- Total Carbohydrate: 40.3 grams carbohydrates
- Saturated Fat: 0.8 grams saturated fat

85. Chinese Spiced Seed Mix

Serving: 2 | Prep: 5mins | Cook: 12mins | Ready in:

Ingredients

- 1 egg white
- 2 tsp Chinese five-spice powder
- ½ tsp salt
- 85g each sunflower and pumpkin seed

Direction

- Heat oven to 150C/130C fan/gas 2. Lightly whisk egg white, then add Chinese five spice and salt. Add sunflower and pumpkin seeds, and coat well. Spread out in a single layer on a lightly oiled baking sheet and bake for 12 mins. Cool before eating.

Nutrition Information

- Calories: 495 calories
- Fiber: 6 grams fiber
- Sugar: 1 grams sugar
- Sodium: 1.4 milligram of sodium
- Total Fat: 40 grams fat
- Total Carbohydrate: 13 grams carbohydrates
- Protein: 21 grams protein
- Saturated Fat: 6 grams saturated fat

86. Crispy Garlic & Rosemary Slices

Serving: 4 | Prep: 15mins | Cook: 25mins | Ready in:

Ingredients

- 4 large potatoes, thinly sliced
- 3 tbsp olive oil
- 2 garlic cloves, sliced
- 1 tbsp rosemaryneedles

Direction

- Heat grill to medium and simmer the potatoes in salted water for 3 mins. Drain well, tip into a shallow baking tray, then gently toss with the oil, garlic, rosemary and seasoning. Spread out in one layer and grill for 10-15 mins or until crisp and golden.

Nutrition Information

- Calories: 245 calories
- Sugar: 1 grams sugar
- Sodium: 0.04 milligram of sodium
- Fiber: 3 grams fiber
- Protein: 5 grams protein
- Total Fat: 9 grams fat
- Saturated Fat: 1 grams saturated fat
- Total Carbohydrate: 39 grams carbohydrates

87. Dried Fruit Energy Nuggets

Serving: Makes 6 | Prep: 10mins | Cook: |Ready in:

Ingredients

- 50g soft dried apricot
- 100g soft dried date
- 50g dried cherry
- 2 tsp coconut oil
- 1 tbsp toasted sesame seed

Direction

- Whizz apricots with dates and cherries in a food processor until very finely chopped. Tip into a bowl and use your hands to work in coconut oil. Shape the mix into walnut-sized balls, then roll in sesame seeds. Store in an airtight container until you need a quick energy fix.

Nutrition Information

- Calories: 113 calories
- Total Carbohydrate: 21 grams carbohydrates
- Sugar: 18 grams sugar
- Fiber: 2 grams fiber
- Protein: 2 grams protein
- Total Fat: 3 grams fat
- Saturated Fat: 1 grams saturated fat

88. Duck Satay With Peanut Sauce

Serving: Makes 20 | Prep: 20mins | Cook: 10mins |Ready in:

Ingredients

- 50g palm or dark brown sugar
- 100ml soy sauce
- 100ml Shaohsing wineor sherry
- 2 star anise
- 1 cinnamon stick
- 1 long red chilli, split down the centre
- 4 skinless duck breasts
- 200g peanut butter
- 4 tbsp vegetable oil

Direction

- Place the sugar, soy, Shaohsing or sherry, star anise, cinnamon, chilli and 100ml water into a pan. Bring to the boil, then remove from the heat and cool. Slice the duck into thin strips, about 5mm wide, and place in the marinade. Leave in the fridge overnight.
- Remove the duck from the marinade. Pour 100ml of the marinade into a small pan along with the peanut butter. Finely chop half the marinated chilli, or pound to a paste using a pestle and mortar, and place in the pan. Cook over a low heat, letting it bubble for at least 5 mins. Add a little water if it starts to dry out. The sauce can be made up to 2 days ahead and kept in the fridge.
- To cook the satay, thread the duck strips onto 20 wooden skewers that have been soaked in water for 1 hr. Mix 4 tbsp of the peanut sauce with the oil and brush all over the duck. Heat a griddle pan until really hot, then cook the duck for about 10 mins, turning until golden all over. You will have to do this in batches, so keep some warm in a low oven or make a day ahead and reheat in the oven. Serve with peanut dipping sauce.

Nutrition Information

- Calories: 125 calories
- Total Fat: 8 grams fat
- Saturated Fat: 2 grams saturated fat
- Total Carbohydrate: 3 grams carbohydrates
- Sugar: 2 grams sugar
- Fiber: 1 grams fiber
- Protein: 9 grams protein
- Sodium: 0.63 milligram of sodium

89. Dukkah Crusted Squash Wedges

Serving: 4 | Prep: 15mins | Cook: 30mins | Ready in:

Ingredients

- 50g blanched hazelnuts
- 1 tbsp coriander seeds
- 2 tbsp sesame seeds
- 1 tbsp ground cumin
- 1 large butternut squash
- 1 tbsp olive oil

Direction

- Heat oven to 200C/180C fan/gas 6. Toast the hazelnuts in a frying pan over a medium heat until golden. Add the coriander and sesame seeds, and toast for 1 min more. Set aside and leave to cool, then add the ground cumin and bash together using a pestle and mortar.
- Peel the butternut squash, remove the seeds and slice into wedges. Toss the wedges with the oil, then mix in the dukkah coating. Spread in a single layer on a baking tray and cook for 30-40 mins, turning halfway through, until tender.

Nutrition Information

- Calories: 282 calories
- Sugar: 15 grams sugar
- Protein: 7 grams protein
- Sodium: 0.1 milligram of sodium
- Total Fat: 14 grams fat
- Fiber: 9 grams fiber
- Saturated Fat: 1 grams saturated fat
- Total Carbohydrate: 28 grams carbohydrates

90. Easy Chicken Casserole

Serving: 4 | Prep: 20mins | Cook: 1hours | Ready in:

Ingredients

- 2 tbsp sunflower oil
- 400g boneless, skinless chicken thigh, trimmed and cut into chunks
- 1 onion, finely chopped
- 3 carrots, finely chopped
- 3 celery sticks, finely chopped
- 2 thyme sprigs or ½ tsp dried
- 1 bay leaf, fresh or dried
- 600ml vegetable or chicken stock
- 2 x 400g / 14oz cans haricot beans, drained
- chopped parsley, to serve

Direction

- Heat the oil in a large pan, add the chicken, then fry until lightly browned. Add the veg, then fry for a few mins more. Stir in the herbs and stock. Bring to the boil. Stir well, reduce the heat, then cover and cook for 40 mins, until the chicken is tender.
- Stir the beans into the pan, then simmer for 5 mins. Stir in the parsley and serve with crusty bread.

Nutrition Information

- Calories: 291 calories
- Protein: 30 grams protein
- Sugar: 9 grams sugar
- Total Carbohydrate: 24 grams carbohydrates
- Saturated Fat: 2 grams saturated fat
- Fiber: 11 grams fiber
- Sodium: 0.66 milligram of sodium
- Total Fat: 9 grams fat

91. John's Great Guacamole

Serving: Serves 4 with leftovers | Prep: | Cook: | Ready in:

Ingredients

- 2 ripe avocados

- 1 lemon, juiced
- 8 drops Tabasco sauce
- 1 long red chilli, deseeded and finely diced
- small bunch coriander, chopped
- small red onion, finely chopped
- 2 tbsp olive oil
- salt, to taste

Direction

- Peel and stone avocados and put in a bowl. Mash using a fork until fairly smooth, but with a little texture. In a small bowl, mix together lemon juice, Tabasco sauce, chilli, coriander, onion, olive oil and salt. Fold this through the avocado. Make it just before serving and don't put it in the fridge.

Nutrition Information

- Calories: 232 calories
- Sugar: 1 grams sugar
- Sodium: 0.08 milligram of sodium
- Total Fat: 24 grams fat
- Total Carbohydrate: 3 grams carbohydrates
- Fiber: 3 grams fiber
- Saturated Fat: 3 grams saturated fat
- Protein: 2 grams protein

92. Lychee & Ginger Sorbet

Serving: 4 | Prep: 20mins | Cook: 5mins |Ready in:

Ingredients

- 2 x 400g cans lychees in syrup
- 2 tsp caster sugar
- thumb-size piece ginger, sliced
- 1 egg white
- 2 pieces stem ginger in syrup, shredded plus some syrup to serve

Direction

- Drain the syrup from two cans of lychees into a small pan. Add the sugar and dissolve over a gentle heat. Bring to the boil for 1 min. Blitz the drained lychees, fresh ginger slices and lychee syrup in a blender until very finely chopped. Pour through a sieve. Tip into a 1-litre container and freeze for at least 6 hrs until solid.
- Break up the frozen mix, then put in a food processor. Tip in the egg white and whizz until thick, pale and smooth. Return to the container and freeze again, ideally overnight. Serve in scoops with slices of stem ginger and syrup poured over, with Chinese fortune cookies or thin butter or almond biscuits.

Nutrition Information

- Calories: 181 calories
- Fiber: 1 grams fiber
- Protein: 2 grams protein
- Sodium: 0.07 milligram of sodium
- Total Carbohydrate: 46 grams carbohydrates
- Sugar: 46 grams sugar

93. Mexican Pork Koftas

Serving: Makes 32 | Prep: 40mins | Cook: 10mins |Ready in:

Ingredients

- 500g minced pork
- 50g fresh white breadcrumbs
- 0.25 - 0.5 tsp hot chilli powder, to taste
- ½ tsp fine sea salt
- finely grated zest 1 lime
- 4 spring onions, finely sliced
- 1 tsp ground turmeric
- 1 tsp ground cumin
- 1 tsp ground coriander
- 3 tbsp finely chopped coriander
- sunflower oil, for greasing
- For the guacamole

- 2 ripe but firm avocados
- 2 garlic cloves, crushed
- 1 red chilli, deseeded and finely chopped
- juice 1 lime
- small pack coriander, chopped

Direction

- Put the pork, breadcrumbs, chilli powder, salt, lime zest, spring onions, turmeric, cumin and ground and chopped coriander in a food processor and season well with ground black pepper. Blitz until the mixture is evenly combined and forms a very thick paste. Form the mince into 32 small ovals and place on a baking tray lined with baking parchment. Can be covered with cling film at this stage and kept in the fridge for up to 8 hrs before baking.
- Heat oven to 220C/200C fan/gas 7. Bake the koftas for 10 mins or until lightly browned and cooked through. To make the guacamole, cut the avocados in half and remove the stones. Scoop the flesh into a bowl and add the garlic, chilli, lime juice and coriander. Mash well with a fork and season, then serve with the hot koftas.

Nutrition Information

- Calories: 46 calories
- Total Fat: 3 grams fat
- Saturated Fat: 1 grams saturated fat
- Total Carbohydrate: 2 grams carbohydrates
- Protein: 3 grams protein
- Sodium: 0.1 milligram of sodium

94. Pea Hummus

Serving: 4 | Prep: 10mins | Cook: |Ready in:

Ingredients

- 200g cooked peas
- 1 garlic clove, crushed

- 1 tbsp tahini
- squeeze of lemon
- 1 tbsp cooked cannellini beans, from a can
- 2 tbsp olive oil
- strips of pitta bread, to serve
- raw vegetable sticks, to serve

Direction

- Blitz all the ingredients together using a hand blender or food processor. Add 1-2 tbsp water, then blitz again. Transfer a portion to a pot and add to a lunchbox with pitta bread strips and veg sticks. Keep the rest chilled for up to 3 days.

Nutrition Information

- Calories: 133 calories
- Protein: 5 grams protein
- Total Fat: 9 grams fat
- Total Carbohydrate: 6 grams carbohydrates
- Sugar: 1 grams sugar
- Sodium: 0.1 milligram of sodium
- Saturated Fat: 1 grams saturated fat
- Fiber: 4 grams fiber

95. Potato Wedges With Curry Sauce

Serving: 6 | Prep: 10mins | Cook: 45mins |Ready in:

Ingredients

- 6 large baking potatoes
- 1 tbsp olive oil
- 2 tbsp tikka masala curry paste
- 1 tbsp tomato purée
- 400g can reduced-fat coconut milk
- handful coriander leaves, chopped (optional)
- juice ½ lemon

Direction

- Heat oven to 200C/fan 180C/gas 6. Cut the potatoes into wedges. Pour the oil into a large roasting pan (no need to peel), toss in the wedges until coated all over, then season with pepper. Bake for 35-40 mins until crisp and golden.
- Put the curry paste and tomato purée in a saucepan, stir well and fry for 1 min. Add the coconut milk, bring to the boil, then gently simmer for 10 mins. Can be frozen or made up to a day ahead. Season to taste and finish with a squeeze of lemon juice and a scattering of coriander, if using.

Nutrition Information

- Calories: 245 calories
- Protein: 5 grams protein
- Sodium: 0.41 milligram of sodium
- Total Carbohydrate: 36 grams carbohydrates
- Sugar: 2 grams sugar
- Saturated Fat: 6 grams saturated fat
- Fiber: 3 grams fiber
- Total Fat: 10 grams fat

96. Red Lentil & Sweet Potato Pâté

Serving: 4 | Prep: | Cook: 30mins | Ready in:

Ingredients

- 1 tbsp olive oil, plus extra for drizzling
- ½ onion, finely chopped
- 1 tsp smoked paprika, plus a little extra
- 1 small sweet potato, peeled and diced
- 140g red lentil
- 3 thyme sprigs, leaves chopped, plus a little extra to decorate (optional)
- 500ml low-sodium vegetable stock (choose a vegan brand, if desired)
- 1 tsp red wine vinegar (choose a vegan brand, if desired)
- pitta bread and vegetable sticks, to serve

Direction

- Heat the oil in a large pan, add the onion and cook slowly until soft and golden. Tip in the paprika and cook for a further 2 mins, then add the sweet potato, lentils, thyme and stock. Bring to a simmer, then cook for 20 mins or until the potato and lentils are tender.
- Add the vinegar and some seasoning, and roughly mash the mixture until you get a texture you like. Chill for 1 hr, then drizzle with olive oil, dust with the extra paprika and sprinkle with thyme sprigs, if you like. Serve with pitta bread and vegetable sticks.

Nutrition Information

- Calories: 200 calories
- Total Carbohydrate: 28 grams carbohydrates
- Protein: 9 grams protein
- Total Fat: 5 grams fat
- Saturated Fat: 1 grams saturated fat
- Sugar: 5 grams sugar
- Sodium: 0.4 milligram of sodium
- Fiber: 3 grams fiber

97. Seeded Flatbreads

Serving: Makes 12 | Prep: 45mins | Cook: 30mins | Ready in:

Ingredients

- 7g sachet dried yeast
- 1 tsp caster sugar
- 400g strong white bread flour
- 200g wholemeal breadflour
- oil, for greasing
- 1 tbsp kalonjiseeds (also called black onion seeds or nigella seeds)
- 2 tbsp sesame seed

Direction

- Mix the yeast with 2 tbsp warm water and sugar, and leave for a few mins. Tip the flours into a large bowl with 1 tsp salt and make a well in the centre. Pour in the yeast mixture and 500ml warm water. Mix with a wooden spoon until it comes together as a dough, then tip onto a work surface and knead for 5-10 mins until smooth and elastic – add a little extra flour if the dough is too sticky. Put the dough in an oiled bowl, cover with a tea towel and leave in a warm place to rise for 1 hr until doubled in size.
- Tip the dough onto your work surface and knock out all the air. Knead the seeds into the dough until well distributed. Divide the dough into 12 pieces, then roll out each as thinly as you can. Heat a large frying pan, cook the flatbreads for 2 mins or until bubbles appear on the surface, then flip over and cook for 2 mins more. Once all are cooked, wrap in foil and keep for up to a day. Pop in a warm oven to reheat.

Nutrition Information

- Calories: 189 calories
- Total Fat: 3 grams fat
- Total Carbohydrate: 34 grams carbohydrates
- Sugar: 1 grams sugar
- Fiber: 3 grams fiber
- Protein: 7 grams protein
- Sodium: 0.4 milligram of sodium

98. Spanish Sardines On Toast

Serving: Serves 2 | Prep: 5mins | Cook: 5mins | Ready in:

Ingredients

- 1 tbsp olive oil
- 1 garlic clove, chopped
- 1 red chilli, deseeded and chopped
- 1 lemon, zest and juice
- 2 x 120g cans sardines in sunflower oil, drained
- 4 slices brown bread
- half small bunch parsley, chopped

Direction

- Heat the olive oil in a frying pan, then sizzle the garlic clove and red chilli. Add the lemon zest.
- Add the sardines and heat through for a few mins until warm.
- Toast the brown bread. Stir the parsley into the sardines, add a squeeze of lemon juice, then divide between the toast and serve.

Nutrition Information

- Calories: 420 calories
- Protein: 29 grams protein
- Total Fat: 21 grams fat
- Total Carbohydrate: 31 grams carbohydrates
- Sugar: 3 grams sugar
- Saturated Fat: 4 grams saturated fat
- Fiber: 3 grams fiber
- Sodium: 1.81 milligram of sodium

99. Spiced Apple Crisps

Serving: 1 | Prep: 5mins | Cook: 1hours | Ready in:

Ingredients

- 2 Granny Smiths
- cinnamon, for sprinkling

Direction

- Heat the oven to 160C/ 140C fan/ gas mark 3. Core the apple and slice through the equator into very thin slices 1 - 2mm thick. Dust with cinnamon and lay flat on a baking sheet lined with parchment paper.
- Cook for 45 mins – 1 hour, turning halfway through and removing any crisps that have

turned brown. Continue cooking until the apples have dried out and are light golden. Cool, store in an airtight container and enjoy as a snack.

Nutrition Information

- Calories: 90 calories
- Sugar: 22 grams sugar
- Fiber: 3.3 grams fiber
- Protein: 0.8 grams protein
- Total Fat: 0.3 grams fat
- Total Carbohydrate: 22 grams carbohydrates

100. Spiced Kale Crisps

Serving: Serves 4-6 as a snack | Prep: 5mins | Cook: 20mins | Ready in:

Ingredients

- 100g chunky chopped kale, or kale leaves, tough stalks removed (weight without stalks)
- ½ tbsp olive oil
- 1 heaped tsp ras el hanout

Direction

- Heat oven to 150C/130C fan/gas 2 and line 2 baking trays with baking parchment. Wash the kale and dry thoroughly. Place in a large bowl, tearing any large leaves into smaller pieces. Drizzle over the oil, then massage into the kale. Sprinkle over the ras el hanout and some sea salt, mix well, then tip onto the trays and spread out in a single layer. Bake for 18-22 mins or until crisp but still green, then leave to cool for a few mins.

Nutrition Information

- Calories: 22 calories
- Total Fat: 1 grams fat
- Total Carbohydrate: 2 grams carbohydrates

- Protein: 1 grams protein
- Sodium: 0.1 milligram of sodium

101. Spicy Bean & Corn Dip

Serving: 4 | Prep: 10mins | Cook: | Ready in:

Ingredients

- 395g can kidney beanin chilli sauce
- 400g can mixed bean, drained
- 326g can sweetcorn, drained
- small red onion, chopped
- 1 red chilli, deseeded and chopped
- small bunch coriander, chopped
- 350g vegetable sticks and tortilla chip, to serve

Direction

- In a food processor, whizz threequarters of the kidney beans and half the mixed beans until smooth. Tip into a bowl and add the remaining ingredients with some seasoning. Serve with crunchy vegetable sticks and tortilla chips for dipping.

Nutrition Information

- Calories: 128 calories
- Total Fat: 1 grams fat
- Total Carbohydrate: 19 grams carbohydrates
- Sugar: 7 grams sugar
- Fiber: 8 grams fiber
- Protein: 8 grams protein
- Sodium: 2.4 milligram of sodium

102. Sweet & Spicy Nuts

Serving: 6 | Prep: 15mins | Cook: 20mins | Ready in:

Ingredients

- 1 tbsp sunflower oil
- 1 tsp ground cinnamon
- ½ tsp mixed spice
- 400g mixed nut, try almonds, Brazil nuts and cashews
- 2 tbsp honey

Direction

- Heat oven to 140C/120C fan/gas 1. Mix the oil with the spices, then stir in the nuts and drizzle over half the honey. Spread over a baking sheet and cook for 10 mins.
- Remove from the oven and drizzle over the remaining honey, then return to the oven and cook for a further 10 mins. Allow to cool completely.

Nutrition Information

- Calories: 449 calories
- Sodium: 0.02 milligram of sodium
- Fiber: 3 grams fiber
- Total Fat: 40 grams fat
- Total Carbohydrate: 11 grams carbohydrates
- Saturated Fat: 6 grams saturated fat
- Sugar: 6 grams sugar
- Protein: 12 grams protein

103. Sweet & Spicy Popcorn

Serving: 2 | Prep: 5mins | Cook: 2mins |Ready in:

Ingredients

- 100g bag salted microwave popcorn
- ¼ tsp chilli powder
- ½ tsp cinnamon
- 1 tbsp agave syrup

Direction

- Cook the microwave popcorn according to the packet instructions. Tip into a large bowl. Sprinkle over the spices, then pour over the

agave syrup. Stir and serve warm or pour into a bag and take to work as an afternoon snack.

Nutrition Information

- Calories: 275 calories
- Protein: 3.8 grams protein
- Sodium: 0.9 milligram of sodium
- Sugar: 9 grams sugar
- Total Fat: 13.6 grams fat
- Total Carbohydrate: 35.1 grams carbohydrates
- Fiber: 5 grams fiber
- Saturated Fat: 6 grams saturated fat

Chapter 5: Dairy-Free Cake Recipes

***

104. Better Beetroot Brownies

Serving: 12 | Prep: 15mins | Cook: 45mins |Ready in:

Ingredients

- 500g whole raw beetroot, washed
- 100ml rapeseed oil
- 250g good-quality dark chocolate (70% cocoa, dairy-free if you want, chopped)
- 3 large eggs
- 200g golden caster sugar
- 2 tsp vanilla extract
- 140g plain flour
- 75g cocoa powder
- 1 tsp baking powder
- 50g walnut piece, roughly chopped
- For the icing
- 100g icing sugar
- 1 tbsp beetroot juice

Direction

- Heat oven to 180C/160C fan/gas 4. Grease and line a 20 x 30cm cake tin with baking parchment. Boil the beetroots in a pan of boiling salted water for 15-20 mins or until tender. Drain and leave to cool before peeling (wear clean rubber gloves to peel if you want to avoid beet-stained hands). Chop one-third of the cooked beetroots into small cubes and blitz the remainder in a blender or food processor to a paste. Sit the paste in a sieve over a bowl – just until you have collected 1-2 tbsp juice. Save this for the icing, and mix the oil into the purée.
- Melt the chocolate slowly in a heatproof bowl over a pan of barely simmering water and leave to cool slightly. Use an electric whisk to beat the eggs, sugar and vanilla together in a large mixing bowl until light, fluffy and tripled in size. Carefully fold the eggs into the beetroot mixture, followed by the melted chocolate. Fold in the flour, cocoa powder and baking powder, then add walnuts and the chopped beetroot.
- Pour into your prepared tin and bake for 20-25 mins. The brownies should still be slightly gooey in the middle. Allow to cool. Mix enough reserved beetroot juice with the icing sugar to get a runny icing – dilute with water if you need. Remove brownies from the tin, drizzle with the icing and cut into squares.

Nutrition Information

- Calories: 408 calories
- Sugar: 41 grams sugar
- Fiber: 3 grams fiber
- Sodium: 0.4 milligram of sodium
- Saturated Fat: 6 grams saturated fat
- Total Carbohydrate: 50 grams carbohydrates
- Total Fat: 20 grams fat
- Protein: 7 grams protein

---

105.   Blueberry & Coconut Cake

Serving: 12 | Prep: 20mins | Cook: 1hours15mins | Ready in:

Ingredients

- 250ml rice bran oil, plus extra for the tin
- 3 eggs
- 225g caster sugar
- 2 tsp vanilla extract
- 300g self-raising flour
- 50g desiccated coconut
- 175ml soya milk
- 140g fresh or frozen blueberries, plus extra to serve
- icing sugar, to dust

Direction

- Heat oven to 180C/160C fan/gas 4 and grease a 22cm Bundt or ring tin. Whisk the oil, eggs, sugar and vanilla in a large bowl. Combine the flour and coconut. Alternately, fold the flour mix and soya milk into the wet ingredients, starting and ending with the flour.
- Spoon a quarter into the tin. Fold the blueberries into the remaining batter, then spoon into the tin. Bake for 1-1¼ hrs, or until a skewer comes out clean. Cover the cake with foil if it browns too quickly.
- Cool in tin for 10 mins, then turn out onto a wire rack and cool completely. Fill centre of the cake with extra blueberries and dust with icing sugar to serve.

Nutrition Information

- Calories: 387 calories
- Total Fat: 24 grams fat
- Sugar: 22 grams sugar
- Fiber: 2 grams fiber
- Sodium: 0.3 milligram of sodium
- Total Carbohydrate: 47 grams carbohydrates
- Protein: 5 grams protein
- Saturated Fat: 7 grams saturated fat

106.   Carrot Cake

Serving: 15 slices | Prep: 1hours15mins | Cook: |Ready in:

Ingredients

- 175g light muscovado sugar
- 175ml sunflower oil
- 3 large eggs, lightly beaten
- 140g grated carrot (about 3 medium)
- 100g raisins
- 1 large orange, zested
- 175g self-raising flour
- 1 tsp bicarbonate of soda
- 1 tsp ground cinnamon
- ½ tsp grated nutmeg (freshly grated will give you the best flavour)
- For the frosting
- 175g icing sugar
- 1½-2 tbsp orange juice

Direction

- Heat the oven to 180C/160C fan/gas 4. Oil and line the base and sides of an 18cm square cake tin with baking parchment.
- Tip the sugar, sunflower oil and eggs into a big mixing bowl. Lightly mix with a wooden spoon. Stir in the carrots, raisins and orange zest.
- Sift the flour, bicarbonate of soda, cinnamon and nutmeg into the bowl. Mix everything together, the mixture will be soft and almost runny.
- Pour the mixture into the prepared tin and bake for 40-45 mins or until it feels firm and springy when you press it in the centre.
- Cool in the tin for 5 mins, then turn it out, peel off the paper and cool on a wire rack. (You can freeze the cake at this point if you want to serve it at a later date.)
- Beat the icing sugar and orange juice in a small bowl until smooth – you want the icing about as runny as single cream. Put the cake on a serving plate and boldly drizzle the icing back and forth in diagonal lines over the top, letting it drip down the sides.

Nutrition Information

- Calories: 265 calories
- Saturated Fat: 2 grams saturated fat
- Sodium: 0.4 milligram of sodium
- Sugar: 24.8 grams sugar
- Protein: 3 grams protein
- Total Carbohydrate: 39 grams carbohydrates
- Fiber: 1 grams fiber
- Total Fat: 12 grams fat

107.   Choc Cherry Fudge Torte With Cherry Sorbet

Serving: Cuts into 10 slices | Prep: 25mins | Cook: 45mins | Ready in:

Ingredients

- 100g dried sour cherry
- 5 tbsp brandy
- 300g gluten- and wheat-free plain flour (we used Doves Farm)
- 85g cocoa, plus extra for dusting
- 200g light soft brown sugar
- 1 tsp gluten-free baking powder
- 1 tsp gluten-free bicarbonate of soda
- 1 tsp xanthan gum
- 150ml sunflower oil
- 350ml rice milk (preferably unsweetened)
- 150ml agave syrup
- a little icing sugar, for dusting
- For the sorbet
- 2 x 600g jars cherry compote
- 200g caster sugar

Direction

- For the sorbet, whizz the compote with the sugar until smooth-ish, then tip into a freezer-proof container. Freeze until solid.
- Mix the cherries and the brandy and leave to soak for a few hrs.
- Heat oven to 160C/140C fan/gas 3. Line the base of a round, 20cm loosebottomed tin with baking parchment. Mix the flour, cocoa, brown sugar, baking powder, bicarb and xanthan gum in a big bowl. Whisk the oil, rice milk and agave syrup, then add to the dry ingredients and stir in with a wooden spoon. Add the cherries and any brandy, then scrape into the tin. Bake for 35-45 mins until crisp on top but fudgy in the centre. Cool in the tin.
- Carefully lift the torte onto a serving plate. Dust with cocoa and icing sugar, and serve with the cherry sorbet.

Nutrition Information

- Calories: 582 calories
- Fiber: 3 grams fiber
- Saturated Fat: 3 grams saturated fat
- Protein: 4 grams protein
- Sodium: 0.7 milligram of sodium
- Total Carbohydrate: 101 grams carbohydrates
- Total Fat: 18 grams fat
- Sugar: 71 grams sugar

---

108.   Chocolate, Orange & Hazelnut Cake

Serving: 10 | Prep: 50mins | Cook: 50mins | Ready in:

Ingredients

- 175ml light-coloured olive oil, plus extra for greasing
- 140g blanched hazelnuts
- 100ml orange juice, plus zest 1 orange
- 140g self-raising flour
- ½ tsp baking powder
- 50g cocoa powder
- 3 large eggs
- 175g light brown muscovado sugar
- For the candied orange slices
- 300g golden caster sugar
- 1 large orange, cut into 3mm/1/8in slices
- To decorate
- 75ml orange juice
- 100g dairy-free dark chocolate
- 50g blanched hazelnuts, toasted
- 1 tsp edible gold powder (see tip)

Direction

- Make the candied orange slices a day ahead if you can. Put the sugar and 300ml water in a medium saucepan and bring to the boil. Reduce to a gentle simmer, add the orange slices and cook for 1 hr-1 hr 10 mins or until the pith is translucent, turning occasionally. Line a baking tray with parchment. Carefully remove the slices from the syrup, place on the prepared tray and set aside to dry (at least 8 hrs) before cutting in half. Reserve the syrup.
- Heat oven to 180C/160C fan/gas 4. Lightly grease a loaf tin (mine was 900g) with olive oil and line with a strip of baking parchment.
- Grind the hazelnuts in a food processor until they resemble coarse breadcrumbs (do not blitz them too much or they will become oily), then add to a bowl along with the orange zest, a pinch of salt and the flour, baking powder and cocoa. Mix together until evenly combined.
- Pour the oil and the orange juice into a jug and mix together. Put the eggs and sugar in a tabletop mixer or large bowl and whisk together for 5-10 mins or until the mixture has tripled in volume and holds a ribbon on the surface when the beaters are lifted out. Slowly pour the oil mixture into the egg mixture and fold together until combined.
- Add the flour mixture to the egg mixture in 3 or 4 additions, folding together until combined. You can't sieve this mixture over the eggs because of the hazelnuts, but try not to dump the flour in one place – you need to be careful and fold the batter to retain its

lightness. Once fully combined, pour the batter into the prepared loaf tin and bake for 50-55 mins or until a skewer inserted into the centre of the cake comes out clean.

- Prick the top of the cake all over, then pour over 5 tbsp of the reserved orange syrup. Cool in the tin for 15 mins, then turn out onto a wire rack to cool completely. Trim the top of the cake (keep this for a mini trifle) and turn out, cut-side down, onto a serving platter.
- To decorate, pour the orange juice into a small pan and bring to a simmer. Put the chocolate in a small bowl, pour the orange juice over and stir together to form a smooth ganache. Set aside in the fridge until thickened, about 20-25 mins. Tip the hazelnuts into a small bowl and add the gold powder with a dash of water, stirring together to coat. Put the ganache in a piping bag fitted with a small round piping tip. Pipe in peaks over the top of the cake, decorating with the golden hazelnuts and the orange slices. Will keep for up to 3 days in an airtight container.

Nutrition Information

- Calories: 635 calories
- Protein: 9 grams protein
- Saturated Fat: 7 grams saturated fat
- Total Fat: 37 grams fat
- Fiber: 4 grams fiber
- Total Carbohydrate: 65 grams carbohydrates
- Sugar: 53 grams sugar
- Sodium: 0.4 milligram of sodium

---

109. Easy Vegan Chocolate Cake

Serving: 16 | Prep: 30mins | Cook: 25mins | Ready in:

Ingredients

- For the cake

- a little dairy-free sunflower spread, for greasing
- 1 large ripe avocado (about 150g)
- 300g light muscovado sugar
- 350g gluten-free plain flour
- 50g good-quality cocoa powder
- 1 tsp bicarbonate of soda
- 2 tsp gluten-free baking powder
- 400ml unsweetened soya milk
- 150ml vegetable oil
- 2 tsp vanilla extract
- For the frosting
- 85g ripe avocado flesh, mashed
- 85g dairy-free sunflower spread
- 200g dairy-free chocolate, 70% cocoa, broken into chunks
- 25g cocoa powder
- 125ml unsweetened soya milk
- 200g icing sugar, sifted
- 1 tsp vanilla extract
- gluten-free and vegan sprinkles, to decorate

Direction

- Heat oven to 160C/140C fan/gas 3. Grease two 20cm sandwich tins with a little dairy-free sunflower spread, then line the bases with baking parchment.
- Put 1 large avocado and 300g light muscovado sugar in a food processor and whizz until smooth.
- Add 350g gluten-free plain flour, 50g cocoa powder, 1 tsp bicarbonate of soda, 2 tsp gluten-free baking powder, 400ml unsweetened soya milk, 150ml vegetable oil and 2 tsp vanilla extract to the bowl with ½ tsp fine salt and process again to a velvety, liquid batter.
- Divide between the tins and bake for 25 mins or until fully risen and a skewer inserted into the middle of the cakes comes out clean.
- Cool in the tins for 5 mins, then turn the cakes onto a rack to cool completely.
- While you wait, start preparing the frosting. Beat together 85g ripe avocado flesh and 85g dairy-free sunflower spread with electric

beaters until creamy and smooth. Pass through a sieve and set aside.

- Melt 200g dairy-free chocolate, either over a bowl of water or in the microwave, then let it cool for a few mins.
- Sift 25g cocoa powder into a large bowl. Bring 125ml unsweetened soya milk to a simmer, then gradually beat into the cocoa until smooth. Cool for a few mins.
- Tip in the avocado mix, 200g sifted icing sugar, melted chocolate and 1 tsp vanilla, and keep mixing to make a shiny, thick frosting. Use this to sandwich and top the cake.
- Cover with sprinkles or your own decoration, then leave to set for 10 mins before slicing. Can be made 2 days ahead.

Nutrition Information

- Calories: 452 calories
- Fiber: 3 grams fiber
- Total Fat: 24 grams fat
- Total Carbohydrate: 53 grams carbohydrates
- Sodium: 0.9 milligram of sodium
- Saturated Fat: 6 grams saturated fat
- Protein: 4 grams protein
- Sugar: 34 grams sugar

110.   Gingered Rich Fruit Cake

Serving: 12 | Prep: 30mins | Cook: 2hours30mins | Ready in:

Ingredients

- oil, for greasing
- 100g each dried currant, sultanas and raisins
- 225g each semi-dried fig and prunes, roughly chopped
- 200g tub crystallised ginger
- 100g stem ginger, from a jar, chopped
- 2 tbsp stem ginger syrup
- 4 tbsp Cointreau
- 1 tsp each ground ginger and mixed spice

- zest 2 lemons
- 150ml olive oil
- 175g light muscovado sugar
- 4 eggs
- 225g gluten-free flour
- 1 tsp gluten-free baking powder
- For the topping
- 4 tbsp apricot jam
- 1 tbsp Cointreau
- 450g mixed fruit, including figs, prunes, date and apricots

Direction

- Heat oven to 140C/fan 120C/gas 1. Lightly oil a 7 1/2cm deep, 25cm round cake tin, and line it with a double layer of baking parchment.
- Mix the dried fruits, ginger and syrup, Cointreau, spices and lemon zest. Put the olive oil, sugar and eggs in a bowl, whisk together until light and fluffy. Sift the flour and baking powder into the mixture and tip in the fruit. Fold and stir together well.
- Spoon the mixture into the cake tin. Bake in the centre of the oven for 2-2 1/2 hrs, or until a skewer inserted into the centre comes out clean. Cover with foil if the cake begins to over-brown. Take from the oven and leave to cool in the tin. Remove, leaving the baking parchment in place until you decorate.
- For the topping: warm the jam and Cointreau together until the jam is liquid, allow to cool. Arrange the fruit on the cake and brush with the jam.

Nutrition Information

- Calories: 600 calories
- Total Fat: 18 grams fat
- Total Carbohydrate: 107 grams carbohydrates
- Fiber: 4 grams fiber
- Protein: 7 grams protein
- Sodium: 0.33 milligram of sodium
- Saturated Fat: 3 grams saturated fat
- Sugar: 43 grams sugar

111.   Sugar Free Carrot Cake

Serving: Cuts into 6-8 slices | Prep: 15mins | Cook: 1hours10mins | Ready in:

Ingredients

- 100g pecan
- 140g self-raising flour, sieved
- 2 tsp ground cinnamon
- 1 tsp bicarbonate of soda
- 140g xylitol
- 2 large eggs (at room temperature)
- 140ml rapeseed oil
- 175g grated carrot
- 100g sultana
- To serve
- drizzle of agave syrup (optional)

Direction

- Preheat the oven to 180C/ 160C fan/ Gas mark 4. Grease and line an 18cm round cake tin with baking parchment. Set aside 12 pecans and roughly chop the rest.
- In a large bowl, mix together the flour, cinnamon, bicarbonate of soda, xylitol and chopped pecans.
- In a separate bowl or jug, beat the eggs and rapeseed oil together. Pour into the flour mixture and stir until combined. Stir through the carrot and sultanas. Spoon into the lined tin, smooth the surface and press whole pecans to form a circle around the edge.
- Cook for 1 hour - 1 hour 10 mins until the top feels springy to the touch and a skewer inserted into the cake comes out clean. Check after 50 mins, if the cake is becoming too dark, cover loosely with foil. Cool on a wire rack for 10 minutes, then turn out and allow to cool. Serve slightly warm or cold. This cake keeps for up to five days in a tin. Before serving, drizzle with agave syrup if you have a sweet tooth.

Nutrition Information

- Calories: 404 calories
- Total Carbohydrate: 40 grams carbohydrates
- Sugar: 10.5 grams sugar
- Protein: 4.8 grams protein
- Sodium: 0.5 milligram of sodium
- Saturated Fat: 2.4 grams saturated fat
- Fiber: 2.2 grams fiber
- Total Fat: 28.2 grams fat

112.   Vegan Carrot Cake

Serving: 15 | Prep: 35mins | Cook: 30mins | Ready in:

Ingredients

- For the icing
- 4 sachets (200g) creamed coconut
- 1 tbsp lemon juice
- 2 tbsp cashew nut butter
- 50g icing sugar
- 60ml oat milk
- For the cake
- 250ml jar coconut oil, melted
- 300g light brown sugar
- 1 ½ tsp vanilla essence
- 210ml dairy free milk, we used oat milk
- 420g plain flour
- 1 ½ tsp baking powder
- 1 ½ tsp bicarbonate of soda
- 1 tsp cinnamon, plus extra cinnamon to decorate
- 1 tsp ginger
- 1 tsp ground nutmeg
- 1 orange, zest only
- 4 medium carrots, grated (you want 270g grated weight)
- 75g chopped walnuts, plus extra to decorate
- edible flowers (optional)

Direction

- Start by making the icing first. Mash the coconut cream with 2 tbsp hot water and the lemon juice until smooth. Add the cashew butter then whisk in the icing sugar followed by the oat milk. Continue to whisk until fully combined, set aside in the fridge until needed.

- Heat the oven to 180C/160C fan/gas mark 4. Grease 2 x 20cm cake tins with a little of the melted coconut oil and line the bases with baking parchment. Whisk together the oil and sugar, then add the vanilla and milk. Combine the flour, baking powder, bicarbonate of soda, spices and orange zest in a separate bowl. Add these to the wet mixture and stir well. Finally stir in the carrot and the nuts. Divide the mixture between the prepared tins and bake for 25-30 mins until a skewer inserted into the middle of the cake comes out cleanly. Cool in the tin for 5 mins before transferring to a wire rack to cool completely.

- Sandwich the cakes together with half the icing then cover the top with the remaining icing (add a splash of oat milk if the icing feels too firm). Scatter over the nuts and dust the cake with a little cinnamon and decorate with edible flowers.

Nutrition Information

- Calories: 501 calories
- Total Carbohydrate: 49 grams carbohydrates
- Total Fat: 31 grams fat
- Sugar: 26 grams sugar
- Sodium: 0.45 milligram of sodium
- Fiber: 2 grams fiber
- Protein: 5 grams protein
- Saturated Fat: 23 grams saturated fat

113.   Vegan Cherry & Almond Brownies

Serving: Makes 12 | Prep: 20mins | Cook: 45mins | Ready in:

Ingredients

- 80g vegan margarine, plus extra for greasing
- 2 tbsp ground flaxseed
- 120g dark chocolate
- ½ tsp coffee granules
- 125g self-raising flour
- 70g ground almond
- 50g cocoa powder
- ¼ tsp baking powder
- 250g golden caster sugar
- 1 ½ tsp vanilla extract
- 70g glacé cherry (rinsed and halved)

Direction

- Heat oven to 170C/150C fan/gas 3½. Grease and line a 20cm square tin with baking parchment. Combine the flaxseed with 6 tbsp water and set aside for at least 5 mins.

- In a saucepan, melt the chocolate, coffee and margarine with 60ml water on a low heat. Allow to cool slightly.

- Put the flour, almonds, cocoa, baking powder and 1/4 tsp salt in a bowl and stir to remove any lumps. Using a hand whisk, mix the sugar into the melted chocolate mixture, and beat well until smooth and glossy, ensuring all the sugar is well dissolved. Stir in the flaxseed mixture and vanilla extract, the cherries and then the flour mixture. It will now be very thick. Stir until combined and spoon into the prepared tin. Bake for 35-45 mins until a skewer inserted in the middle comes out clean with moist crumbs. Allow to cool in the tin completely, then cut into squares. Store in an airtight container and eat within 3 days.

Nutrition Information

- Calories: 296 calories
- Protein: 4 grams protein
- Total Carbohydrate: 36 grams carbohydrates
- Saturated Fat: 5 grams saturated fat
- Sodium: 0.2 milligram of sodium
- Total Fat: 15 grams fat
- Sugar: 27 grams sugar
- Fiber: 3 grams fiber

114. Vegan Chocolate Cake

Serving: 12 | Prep: 35mins | Cook: 20mins | Ready in:

Ingredients

- 150g dairy-free spread, plus extra for the tins
- 300ml dairy-free milk, we used oat milk
- 1 tbsp cider vinegar
- 300g self-raising flour
- 200g golden caster sugar
- 4 tbsp cocoa powder
- 1 tsp bicarbonate of soda
- ½ tsp vanilla extract
- For the buttercream
- 100g dairy-free dark chocolate
- 200g dairy-free spread
- 400g icing sugar
- 5 tbsp cocoa powder
- 1 tbsp dairy-free milk, such as oat milk
- To decorate
- handful of fresh, seasonal fruits such as cherries, blackberries or figs

Direction

- Heat oven to 190C/170C fan/gas 5. Grease the base and sides of 2 x 20cm sandwich tins with dairy-free spread, then line the bases with baking parchment.
- Put the dairy-free milk in a jug and add the vinegar – it will split but don't worry. Put all of the other cake ingredients into a large bowl, pour over the milk mixture and beat well until smooth. Divide the mixture between the prepared tins and bake for 25-30 mins or until a skewer inserted into the middle of the cakes comes out cleanly. Leave to cool in the tins for 10mins then turn out onto wire racks to cool completely.
- To make the buttercream, put the chocolate into a heatproof bowl and melt in the microwave, stirring every 30 seconds. Leave the melted chocolate to cool for 5 minutes.
- Beat the dairy-free spread and icing sugar together with a wooden spoon then sift in the cocoa powder with a pinch of salt. Pour in the melted chocolate and dairy-free milk and keep mixing until smooth.
- Sandwich the two cooled sponges together with half of the buttercream then pile the rest on top and down the sides. Decorate with the fresh fruit.

Nutrition Information

- Calories: 606 calories
- Protein: 6 grams protein
- Sodium: 1.2 milligram of sodium
- Saturated Fat: 8 grams saturated fat
- Total Carbohydrate: 75 grams carbohydrates
- Sugar: 53 grams sugar
- Total Fat: 30 grams fat
- Fiber: 4 grams fiber

115. Vegan Cupcakes

Serving: Makes 12 | Prep: 30mins | Cook: 20mins | Ready in:

Ingredients

- 150ml almond or soy milk
- ½ tsp cider vinegar
- 110g vegan butter or sunflower spread
- 110g caster sugar
- 1 tsp vanilla extract
- 110g self-raising flour
- ½ tsp baking powder
- For the buttercream
- 125g vegan butter
- 250g icing sugar
- 1¼ tsp vanilla extract
- a few drops of vegan food colourings (check the label)

Direction

- Heat the oven to 180C/160C fan/gas 4. Line the holes of a 12-hole cupcake tin with paper cases. Stir the milk and vinegar in a jug and leave to thicken slightly for a few mins.
- Beat the butter and sugar with an electric whisk until well combined. Whisk in the vanilla, then add the milk a splash at a time, alternating with spoonfuls of the flour. Fold in any remaining flour, the baking powder and a pinch of salt until you get a creamy batter. Don't worry if it looks a little curdled at this stage.
- Divide between the cupcake cases, filling them two-thirds full, and bake for 20 - 25 mins until golden and risen. Leave to cool on a wire rack.
- To make the buttercream, beat the butter, icing sugar and vanilla with an electric whisk until pale and creamy. Divide between bowls and colour with different food colourings until you get desired strength. Spoon or pipe onto the cooled cupcakes.

Nutrition Information

- Calories: 265 calories
- Saturated Fat: 3 grams saturated fat
- Total Carbohydrate: 37 grams carbohydrates
- Protein: 1 grams protein
- Fiber: 0.4 grams fiber
- Total Fat: 12 grams fat
- Sugar: 30 grams sugar
- Sodium: 0.28 milligram of sodium

116. Vegan Cupcakes With Banana & Peanut Butter

Serving: Makes 16 | Prep: 25mins | Cook: 20mins | Ready in:

Ingredients

- 240g self-raising flour
- 140g golden caster sugar
- 1 tsp bicarbonate of soda
- 240g egg-free mayonnaise
- 2 large or 3 small ripe bananas, mashed
- 1 tsp vanilla extract
- 25g vegan dark chocolate chip
- For the icing
- 80g vegan margarine
- 250g icing sugar
- 25ml vegan milk (we used almond milk)
- 2 tbsp smooth peanut butter

Direction

- Heat oven to 170C/150C fan/gas 3½. Line muffin tins with 16 cases. In a bowl, combine the flour, sugar, ½ tsp salt and bicarbonate of soda. In a second bowl or a jug, mix the mayonnaise, mashed bananas and vanilla extract. Pour the wet ingredients into the dry and mix with a spoon until just combined (don't overmix or your cupcakes will be heavy). Spoon the mixture into the cases and bake for 20 mins.
- When the cupcakes come out of the oven, sprinkle the chocolate chips over – they will melt and then harden again, so don't touch them.
- For the icing, combine the vegan margarine and icing sugar in an electric mixer, then add the vegan milk and continue to mix on a slow speed until completely combined. Turn the mixer up and combine for a further 3 mins. Finally, stir in the peanut butter. Pipe or simply spread the icing on top of the cakes. Store in an airtight container and eat within 2 days.

Nutrition Information

- Calories: 295 calories
- Total Fat: 14 grams fat
- Fiber: 1 grams fiber
- Saturated Fat: 3 grams saturated fat
- Total Carbohydrate: 40 grams carbohydrates
- Sugar: 28 grams sugar
- Protein: 2 grams protein

- Sodium: 0.7 milligram of sodium

117. Vegan Mug Cake

Serving: 1 | Prep: 5mins | Cook: 2mins |Ready in:

Ingredients

- 3 tbsp dairy-free milk, we used oat milk
- pinch lemon zest
- 1 tsp lemon juice
- 1 tbsp sunflower oil
- 4 tbsp self-raising flour
- 2 tbsp caster sugar
- pinch bicarbonate of soda
- 4 fresh or frozen raspberries
- To serve
- coconut cream or dairy-free ice cream

Direction

- Put the milk in a microwave-safe mug, add the lemon zest and juice and leave to sit for 2-3 mins. It should start to look a bit grainy, as if it has split. Stir in the sunflower oil, flour, sugar and bicarbonate of soda. Mix really well with a fork until smooth.
- Drop in the raspberries then microwave on high for 1 min 30 secs, or until puffed up and cooked through.
- Serve with a drizzle of coconut cream, or a scoop of dairy-free ice cream if you like.

Nutrition Information

- Calories: 576 calories
- Total Carbohydrate: 104 grams carbohydrates
- Protein: 8 grams protein
- Total Fat: 13 grams fat
- Fiber: 4 grams fiber
- Sodium: 1.4 milligram of sodium
- Sugar: 43 grams sugar
- Saturated Fat: 2 grams saturated fat

118. Vegan Rhubarb & Custard Bake

Serving: Cuts into 15 squares | Prep: 20mins | Cook: 1hours15mins |Ready in:

Ingredients

- 250g rhubarb, cut into 1in lengths
- 275g golden caster sugar
- 1 tsp vanilla bean paste
- 250g vegan margarine, plus extra for greasing
- 2 tbsp ground flaxseed
- 150g soya custard, plus extra to serve (optional)
- 250g self-raising flour
- 1 tsp baking powder
- 1 tsp vanilla extract
- 130g unsweetened apple sauce
- icing sugar, to serve (optional)

Direction

- Heat oven to 200C/180C fan/gas 6 and put the rhubarb in a roasting tin. Sprinkle over 25g of the caster sugar, add the vanilla bean paste, give the tin a shake and put it in the oven for 15 mins. Remove, pour away any liquid from the tin and leave the rhubarb to cool.
- Reduce oven to 170C/150C fan/gas 31/2. Grease and line a 25 x 20cm cake tin with baking parchment. In a small bowl, mix the flaxseed with 6 tbsp water and set aside for 5 mins.
- In a bowl, beat together the margarine, 100g of the custard, the flour, baking powder, vanilla extract and remaining sugar. Once this is well combined, light and fluffy, add the apple sauce and flaxseed mixture.
- Put a third of the mixture in the tin and top with a third of the rhubarb. Repeat twice more, then dot teaspoons of the remaining custard on top.
- Bake in the oven for 45 mins, then cover with foil and bake for a further 30 mins or until golden brown and a skewer comes out clean

when inserted in the middle. Serve warm as a pudding with soya custard, if you like. Or allow to cool completely, then sprinkle with icing sugar and enjoy as a cake. Eat the same day.

Nutrition Information

- Calories: 274 calories
- Saturated Fat: 3 grams saturated fat
- Protein: 2 grams protein
- Total Fat: 15 grams fat
- Sugar: 21 grams sugar
- Fiber: 2 grams fiber
- Total Carbohydrate: 34 grams carbohydrates
- Sodium: 0.3 milligram of sodium

119. Vegan Sponge Cake

Serving: 10 | Prep: 20mins | Cook: 35mins | Ready in:

Ingredients

- 150g dairy-free spread, plus extra for the tins
- 300ml dairy-free milk, we used oat milk
- 1 tbsp cider vinegar
- 1 vanilla pod, seeds scraped
- 300g self-raising flour
- 200g golden caster sugar
- 1 tsp bicarbonate of soda
- For the filling
- 100g dairy-free spread
- 200g icing sugar, plus extra for dusting
- 4 tbsp jam, we used strawberry

Direction

- Heat oven to 180C/160C fan/gas 4. Line the bases of 2 x 20cm sandwich tins with baking parchment and grease with a little of the dairy-free spread.
- Put the dairy-free milk into a jug and add the vinegar, leave for a few minutes until it looks a little lumpy. Put half of the vanilla seeds and

all the other cake ingredients into a large bowl then pour over the milk mixture. Using electric beaters or a wooden spoon, beat everything together until smooth.

- Divide the mix between your two tins then bake in the centre of the oven for 30-35 mins or until a skewer inserted into the middle of the cakes comes out cleanly. Leave them in their tins until cool enough to handle then carefully turn out onto wire racks to cool completely.
- While the cakes are cooling, make the filling. To make the vegan buttercream, whisk or beat together the dairy-free spread, icing sugar and remaining vanilla seeds until pale and fluffy. Dairy-free spreads do vary so if the spread you are using is quite soft try to avoid using electric beaters. Stir the ingredients together instead to avoid overworking it. However, if the mixture is too firm, use electric beaters to help lighten it and add 1-2 tbsp of dairy-free milk when whisking.
- Spread the jam onto one of the cooled sponges, top with the buttercream then place the other sponge on top. Dust the assembled cake with a little icing sugar or caster sugar before slicing.

Nutrition Information

- Calories: 482 calories
- Saturated Fat: 4 grams saturated fat
- Total Carbohydrate: 69 grams carbohydrates
- Sugar: 45 grams sugar
- Protein: 3 grams protein
- Fiber: 1 grams fiber
- Sodium: 1.2 milligram of sodium
- Total Fat: 21 grams fat

120. Yule Slice

Serving: Cuts into 16 thin slices | Prep: | Cook: 1hours45mins | Ready in:

Ingredients

- 200g walnut halves
- 100g hazelnut
- 50g blanched almond
- 200g raisin
- 100g pitted date, chopped
- 200g dried apricot, chopped
- 140g glacé cherry or pineapple
- 100g plain flour
- 2 tsp mixed spice
- ½ tsp baking powder
- 175g dark muscovado sugar
- 3 eggs
- 1 tsp vanilla extract
- icing sugar, for dusting

Direction

- Heat oven to 150C/fan 130C/gas 2. Line the base and sides of a 1.5-litre loaf tin (a long thin one is best) with baking parchment. Mix the nuts and dried fruit thoroughly in a large bowl using your hands. Sift in the flour, spice and baking powder, then add the sugar and mix everything well. Beat the eggs with the vanilla, then add to the dry mix, turning everything together well until there is no dry mix visible.
- Turn into the prepared tin and smooth the top. Bake for 1½-1¾ hrs, then cool in the tin for 15 mins. Turn out, peel off the paper and cool on a wire rack. Dust the top thickly with icing sugar, to serve.

Nutrition Information

- Calories: 322 calories
- Protein: 7 grams protein
- Total Fat: 16 grams fat
- Total Carbohydrate: 41 grams carbohydrates
- Fiber: 3 grams fiber
- Sodium: 0.15 milligram of sodium
- Saturated Fat: 2 grams saturated fat
- Sugar: 36 grams sugar

Chapter 6: Dairy-Free Dessert Recipes

***

121. Cheat's Pineapple, Thai Basil & Ginger Sorbet

Serving: 6 | Prep: 5mins | Cook: | Ready in:

Ingredients

- 1 large pineapple, peeled, cored and cut into chunks
- juice and zest 1 lime
- 1 small piece of ginger, sliced
- handful Thai basil leaves, plus a few extra little ones to serve
- 75g white caster sugar
- vodka or white rum (optional)

Direction

- A couple of days before eating, tip everything into a blender or smoothie maker with 200ml water and blitz until very smooth. Pour into a freezable container and freeze overnight until solid.
- A few hours before serving, remove from the freezer and allow to defrost slightly so it slides out of the container in a block. Chop the block into ice cube-sized chunks and blitz in the blender or smoothie maker again until you have a thick, slushy purée. Tip back into the container and refreeze for 1 hr or until it can be scooped out.
- To serve, scoop the sorbet into chilled bowls or glasses and top with extra basil. If you want you can drizzle with something a little more potent, such as vodka or white rum.

Nutrition Information

- Calories: 145 calories
- Total Carbohydrate: 33 grams carbohydrates
- Sugar: 33 grams sugar
- Fiber: 3 grams fiber
- Protein: 1 grams protein

122. Cherries In Rosé Wine & Vanilla Syrup

Serving: 4 | Prep: | Cook: 20mins | Ready in:

Ingredients

- 425ml rosé wine
- 1 vanilla pod, split lengthways
- 100g demerara sugar
- 500g cherry

Direction

- Tip the wine into a medium pan, then add the vanilla pod to the pan with the sugar. Bring to the boil, then reduce the heat and simmer until the sugar has dissolved.
- Stone the cherries if you want, or leave them as they are. Add to the pan and cook gently for 6 mins. Remove with a slotted spoon to a bowl. Increase the heat, then boil the liquid for 8-10 mins until slightly syrupy. Pour over the cherries and serve warm or cold in glass bowls.

Nutrition Information

- Calories: 199 calories
- Protein: 1 grams protein
- Sodium: 0.02 milligram of sodium
- Total Carbohydrate: 43 grams carbohydrates
- Sugar: 43 grams sugar
- Fiber: 1 grams fiber

123. Chocolate Crunch & Raspberry Pots

Serving: 4 | Prep: | Cook: 10mins | Ready in:

Ingredients

- 250g punnet raspberry
- 2 tbsp Cointreau (or Grand Marnier)
- zest and juice from 1 small orange
- 100g pack dairy, gluten and wheat-free, 'Free From' chocolate (we used Kinnerton Luxury Dark Chocolate Bar)
- 3 tbsp soya milk
- 50g caster sugar
- 6 tbsp gluten, wheat and nut-free muesli muesli (we used The Food Doctor Cereal, nut-free)

Direction

- Divide the raspberries between 4 glasses. Sprinkle ½ tbsp of Cointreau and a little orange zest and juice over each, then set aside.
- Melt the chocolate and stir into the soya milk, then set aside. Tip the sugar into a pan along with 3 tbsp water. Over a gentle heat, cook without stirring for about 7 mins until the sugar melts and starts to turn golden brown. Tip in the muesli, stir, then pour onto a tray lined with baking parchment. Leave to cool, then shatter into thin shards.
- Divide the chocolate mixture between the glasses and allow to cool, but don't refrigerate. Scatter over the caramel crunch to serve.

Nutrition Information

- Calories: 297 calories
- Fiber: 6 grams fiber
- Total Fat: 11 grams fat
- Saturated Fat: 6 grams saturated fat
- Total Carbohydrate: 43 grams carbohydrates
- Sodium: 0.08 milligram of sodium
- Protein: 5 grams protein
- Sugar: 33 grams sugar

124. Cranberry, Maple & Pecan Pudding

Serving: 8 | Prep: | Cook: 3hours | Ready in:

Ingredients

- 100g each semi-dried prunes and date, stoned and chopped
- 100g each raisins and sultanas
- 100g pack dried cranberry
- 170g gluten-free flour
- 1 tsp gluten-free baking powder
- 100g pack pecan, roughly chopped
- 2 tsp mixed spice
- grated zest and juice of 2 oranges
- 100g dark muscovado sugar
- 5 tbsp maple syrup
- 2 eggs, beaten
- 100ml sunflower oil
- oil, for greasing
- 100g fresh cranberry
- 5 tbsp maple syrup

Direction

- Put all the ingredients for the pudding into a big bowl and stir together until well mixed. Don't be put off by the consistency of the mixture – it is quite wet. Lightly oil a 1.5 litre pudding basin. Tip the mixture into this and press down. Make a cover for the pudding basin using a double layer each of oiled greaseproof paper and aluminium foil. Make a pleat in the middle of these sheets to allow for expansion of the pudding. Press it over the top of the pudding basin and secure it well with a double piece of string. Use a little extra string to make a handle for ease of lifting in and out of the boiling water.
- Cook the pudding in a large pan with a well-fitting lid. There should be enough boiling water to come two-thirds up the sides of the basin at all times – so keep an eye on it. Cook the pudding for 3 hrs.
- To make the topping, cook the cranberries in the maple syrup until they burst open and become syrupy. Once the pudding is cooked, remove the cover and carefully tip it onto a large serving plate. Spoon the hot cranberry and maple syrup over the top and serve straight away.

Nutrition Information

- Calories: 550 calories
- Sodium: 0.3 milligram of sodium
- Sugar: 24 grams sugar
- Fiber: 4 grams fiber
- Saturated Fat: 3 grams saturated fat
- Total Carbohydrate: 86 grams carbohydrates
- Protein: 6 grams protein
- Total Fat: 23 grams fat

125. Creamy Rice With Double Apricots

Serving: 4 | Prep: | Cook: | Ready in:

Ingredients

- 50g pudding rice
- 500ml carton long-life vanilla-flavoured sweetened soya milk alternative (we used UHT Provamel organic vanilla)
- 50g ready-to-eat dried apricots, chopped into small pieces
- 1 tbsp golden caster sugar
- 250ml carton soya single cream alternative (we used UHT Provamel Soya Dream)
- 8 tbsp apricot compote or 4 tbsp apricot conserve
- 1 tbsp shelled pistachio nuts, chopped

Direction

- Put the rice and soya milk into a medium-sized saucepan, stir and bring to the boil. Reduce the heat immediately or the soya will bubble up and can easily boil over. Half cover the pan with a lid then cook gently for 40-45 minutes over a very low heat, stirring occasionally until the rice has swollen and is very tender. The mixture should be thick and creamy.

- While the rice is cooking, mix together the apricots, sugar and single cream alternative.
- Remove the rice from the heat, leave to cool for 15 minutes, then stir in the apricot mixture. Spoon into 4 small tumblers or glass dishes. Cover and chill in the fridge for 30 minutes (or longer if you have the time).
- To serve, spoon two tbsp of apricot compote or 1 tbsp of conserve on top of each dessert and scatter the pistachios on top.

Nutrition Information

- Calories: 280 calories
- Sugar: 6 grams sugar
- Fiber: 2 grams fiber
- Sodium: 0.31 milligram of sodium
- Total Fat: 15 grams fat
- Saturated Fat: 1 grams saturated fat
- Total Carbohydrate: 30 grams carbohydrates
- Protein: 8 grams protein

126.   Gluten Free Scones

Serving: Makes 6-8 | Prep: 20mins | Cook: 15mins | Ready in:

Ingredients

- 250g gluten free self-raising flour
- ½ tsp fine salt
- 1 tsp xanthan gum
- 1 tsp gluten-free baking powder
- 50g caster sugar
- 40g cold butter, cubed
- 75ml whole milk
- 1 large egg and 1 egg yolk
- 50g sultanas (optional)

Direction

- Mix the flour, salt, xanthan gum, baking powder and sugar together in a bowl. Rub in the butter with your fingertips until you have fine breadcrumbs. You can also do this by gradually pulsing the mixture in a food processor until it resembles breadcrumbs.
- Whisk together the milk and whole egg and gradually mix into the flour mixture with your hands until you have a smooth dough. Mix in the sultanas, if using. Knead briefly to come together into a ball.
- Gently roll out the scone dough until 2cm thick. Transfer to a baking tray lined with parchment and chill for 30 mins to firm up the dough – this makes them easier to cut out.
- Remove the dough from the fridge and, using a 5cm cutter, cut out 6-8 scones (press the offcuts together and re-roll when you need to). Put the scones upside down (this will mean you get a neater top when baked) onto another baking tray lined with baking parchment, spread 2cm apart.
- Whisk the egg yolk and evenly brush the tops of the scones, making sure that the egg wash doesn't run down the sides of the scones otherwise they will rise unevenly. Put the scones on a tray and transfer to the freezer for 15 mins. Heat oven to 220C/200C fan/gas 7. Remove the scones from the freezer and brush the tops with the beaten egg again, then bake for 12-15 mins until golden brown. Eat just warm or cold, generously topped with jam and cream, if you like.

Nutrition Information

- Calories: 193 calories
- Fiber: 1 grams fiber
- Protein: 4 grams protein
- Total Fat: 6 grams fat
- Sugar: 7 grams sugar
- Sodium: 0.82 milligram of sodium
- Saturated Fat: 3 grams saturated fat
- Total Carbohydrate: 30 grams carbohydrates

127. Instant Berry Banana Slush

Serving: 2 | Prep: 5mins | Cook: | Ready in:

Ingredients

- 2 ripe bananas
- 200g frozen berry mix (blackberries, raspberries and currants)

Direction

- Slice the bananas into a bowl and add the frozen berry mix. Blitz with a stick blender to make a slushy ice and serve straight away in two glasses with spoons.

Nutrition Information

- Calories: 119 calories
- Protein: 2 grams protein
- Total Fat: 0.4 grams fat
- Saturated Fat: 0.1 grams saturated fat
- Total Carbohydrate: 24 grams carbohydrates
- Sugar: 22 grams sugar
- Fiber: 5 grams fiber

128. Lemon Sorbet

Serving: 6 | Prep: 10mins | Cook: 10mins | Ready in:

Ingredients

- 250g white caster sugar
- thick strip of lemon peel
- juice of 2-3 lemons
- 2 tbsp vodka (optional)
- To serve
- zest of half a lemon

Direction

- Heat 250ml water, the sugar and the lemon peel in a small pan until the sugar has dissolved then bring the mixture to the boil. Cook for 3 mins then turn off the heat and leave to cool. Pick out the lemon peel and discard. Measure out 100ml of lemon juice and add to the sugar mixture along with the vodka if using.
- Pour into a freezer box and freeze for 1hr 30 mins then mix up with a whisk to break up and incorporate the ice crystals (which will be starting to form at the edges) before returning to the freezer.
- Keep mixing the sorbet once an hour for 4 hours to break up the ice crystals. Stop mixing when firm but still scoopable then store in the freezer for up to 1 month. Serve scoops of sorbet decorated with a few curls of lemon zest.

Nutrition Information

- Calories: 179 calories
- Total Carbohydrate: 42 grams carbohydrates
- Sugar: 42 grams sugar

129. Panna Cotta With Apricot Compote

Serving: 4 | Prep: | Cook: 20mins | Ready in:

Ingredients

- 3 level tsp gelatine(or veggie gelatine or agar agar)
- 500ml soya milk (we used So Good)
- zest 1 lemon
- 1 vanilla pod, split
- splash of rum brandy
- 50g golden caster sugar
- 350g ripe apricot
- 50g caster sugar

Direction

- Sprinkle the gelatine onto 3 tbsp water and soak for 5 mins. Scrape the seeds out of the vanilla pod into the pan and put the pod into the milk. Put the soya milk, zest, vanilla pod, sugar and rum into a pan. Heat until the liquid just comes to the boil (if using veggie gelatine, you'll need to bring it to the boil – check pack instructions), then remove from the heat and stir in the gelatine. Cool for 10 mins. If the gelatine clumps together, whisk thoroughly. Strain the milk mixture, then divide between 4 ramekins. Cover and refrigerate until set (approximately 2 hrs).
- Halve and stone the apricots. Put the sugar and 150ml water into a pan, then heat until the sugar has dissolved. Add the apricots and cook over a gentle heat for 12-15 mins or until the apricots are soft, then leave to cool. Serve in a dish alongside the panna cotta.

Nutrition Information

- Calories: 146 calories
- Total Carbohydrate: 36 grams carbohydrates
- Sugar: 26 grams sugar
- Fiber: 2 grams fiber
- Protein: 7 grams protein
- Sodium: 0.14 milligram of sodium
- Total Fat: 2 grams fat

---

130.   Raspberry & Red Wine Slush With Peach Salad

Serving: Serves 4 | Prep: 20mins | Cook: | Ready in:

Ingredients

- 225g punnet raspberries
- 400ml light red wine, such as a Beaujolais or Gamay
- 140g caster sugar
- 2 ripe peaches, halved, stoned and cut into wedges
- handful mintleaves

Direction

- Tip the raspberries, wine and sugar into a blender and blitz until smooth (this can also be done in a large jug with a hand blender). Push the liquid through a sieve to get rid of some of the pips, then churn in an ice-cream machine until the texture of soft sorbet.
- Transfer to a freezable container and freeze for at least 4 hrs. If you don't have an ice-cream machine, freeze the liquid until it starts to become icy, then mash the ice crystals with a fork until slushy. Repeat 3 or 4 times until you have the texture of sorbet.
- To serve, toss the peaches with the mint and serve alongside bowls of the scooped slush.

Nutrition Information

- Calories: 240 calories
- Sodium: 0.03 milligram of sodium
- Total Carbohydrate: 44 grams carbohydrates
- Sugar: 43 grams sugar
- Fiber: 2 grams fiber
- Protein: 2 grams protein

---

131.   Rhubarb & Star Anise Sorbet

Serving: Makes about 500ml | Prep: 20mins | Cook: 20mins | Ready in:

Ingredients

- 700g thin forced rhubarb, trimmed, rinsed and cut into 2cm/ 3/4 in-long pieces
- 140g golden caster sugar
- 3 tbsp liquid glucose (I used Dr Oetker)
- 1 vanilla pod
- 2 star anise
- juice 1 lemon
- 1 tbsp vodka (optional)

Direction

- Put the rhubarb in a saucepan and add the sugar, 75ml water and the liquid glucose. Scrape the seeds from the vanilla pod and add to the pan (with the pod) along with the star anise.
- Place over a medium-high heat and bring to the boil, stirring occasionally. Reduce the heat slightly and cook for 15 mins until the sugar has dissolved and the fruit is soft and starting to break down. Remove from the heat and fish out the vanilla pod and star anise. Purée in a blender.
- Pour the mixture through a fine mesh strainer, removing any remaining stringy bits of rhubarb. Transfer to a jug and stir in the lemon juice and vodka, if using. Cover and put in the fridge until fully chilled before churning in an ice cream machine, according to the manufacturer's instructions. Scrape the sorbet into an airtight container and freeze for at least 3 hrs before serving. Will keep, frozen, for up to 1 month.

Nutrition Information

- Calories: 100 calories
- Sugar: 20 grams sugar
- Fiber: 2 grams fiber
- Protein: 1 grams protein
- Total Carbohydrate: 23 grams carbohydrates

---

132.   Salted Caramel Biscuit Bars

Serving: makes 18 | Prep: 45mins | Cook: 15mins | Ready in:

Ingredients

- For the biscuit base
- 80g porridge oats
- 20g ground almonds
- 50ml maple syrup
- 3 tbsp coconut oil, melted
- For the caramel filling
- 125g medjool dates, pitted
- 1 ½ tbsp smooth peanut butter or almond butter
- 2 tbsp coconut oil, melted
- ½ tbsp almond milk
- generous pinch of salt
- For the topping
- 150g dairy-free dark chocolate

Direction

- Heat oven to 180C/160C fan/gas 4 and line a large baking tray with baking parchment.
- For the base, blitz the oats in a food processor until flour-like. Add the remaining ingredients and whizz until the mixture starts to clump together. Scrape into a bowl, then roll and cut into 18 equal-sized rectangular bars, about 9 x 2cm. Place on the prepared tray and use a small palette knife to neaten the tops and sides of each biscuit. Bake for about 10 mins until lightly golden at the edges, then leave to cool.
- Meanwhile, put all the caramel ingredients in the food processor (no need to rinse it first) and blitz until it forms smooth, shiny clumps. Using a spatula, push the mixture together, then roll into 18 even-sized balls using your hands.
- Once the biscuits are cool, squash the caramel onto them. Use your fingers to press it into shape and smooth out any bumps, especially around the edges (as they will show underneath the chocolate coating).
- Melt the chocolate in a heatproof bowl set over a pan of simmering water – make sure the water doesn't touch the bowl (otherwise, it might seize and go grainy). Carefully dip one of the caramel-coated biscuits in the chocolate, turning it gently with a small palette knife (use this to lift it out as well). Use a spoon to drizzle over more chocolate to coat it fully. Let the excess chocolate drip into the bowl, then carefully put the biscuit back on the lined tray.
- Repeat with the remaining biscuits, then chill in the fridge for at least 30 mins or until the chocolate has set. Put the biscuits in an airtight

container and store in the fridge. Will keep for five days.

Nutrition Information

- Calories: 137 calories
- Sodium: 0.1 milligram of sodium
- Total Fat: 8 grams fat
- Sugar: 8 grams sugar
- Fiber: 2 grams fiber
- Protein: 2 grams protein
- Total Carbohydrate: 13 grams carbohydrates
- Saturated Fat: 5 grams saturated fat

133.   Strawberry & Rose Sorbet

Serving: Serves 6 (makes about 1.5 litres) | Prep: 10mins | Cook: 5mins | Ready in:

Ingredients

- 300g caster sugar
- 900g ripe strawberry, hulled
- juice 1 lemon
- 2 tsp - 2tbsp (depending on strength) rosewater
- handful pink rosépetals, to serve (optional)

Direction

- In a medium pan, combine the sugar with 300ml water. Let the sugar dissolve, then bring to the boil for 1 min. Put the strawberries in a blender or food processor and pulse until smooth. Trickle in the sugar syrup, blend again, then add the lemon juice and rose water.
- Pour the strawberry mixture into a large freezer-proof container (an old ice cream tub is perfect), then freeze until almost solid, mashing in the ice crystals every 1-2 hrs until the sorbet is thick and smooth. Wrap well and freeze until solid. Allow to soften for 15 mins before scooping. Best eaten within a month.

Nutrition Information

- Calories: 238 calories
- Sugar: 58 grams sugar
- Fiber: 2 grams fiber
- Protein: 1 grams protein
- Total Carbohydrate: 58 grams carbohydrates

134.   Tropical Punch Cups

Serving: 10 | Prep: 15mins | Cook: | Ready in:

Ingredients

- ½ fresh pineapple, cut into chunks
- 2 mangoes, peeled and cut into chunks
- 2 starfruit, sliced
- 150ml guavajuice (or other tropical fruit juice)
- 50ml gingerbeer

Direction

- Mix together all the fruit in a large bowl with the guava juice, then chill until ready to serve. At the last minute, pour over the ginger beer and serve with small cups or bowls on the side for spooning the drinks and fruit into.

Nutrition Information

- Calories: 83 calories
- Total Carbohydrate: 20 grams carbohydrates
- Sugar: 20 grams sugar
- Protein: 1 grams protein
- Sodium: 0.01 milligram of sodium

135.   Vegan Eton Mess

Serving: 4 | Prep: 20mins | Cook: 1hours30mins | Ready in:

Ingredients

- Drained liquid from a 400g can chickpeas (aquafaba)
- 100g golden caster sugar
- 500g mixed berries
- 2 tbsp icing sugar
- ½ tbsp rose water
- 400ml vegan coconut yogurt (we used COYO, vanilla flavoured)
- rose petals, to serve

Direction

- Heat oven to 110C/90C fan/gas 1 and line a baking tray with parchment. Whisk the drained chickpea liquid with an electric whisk until white, fluffy and just holding its shape – be persistent, this will take longer than you imagine. Gradually whisk in the caster sugar until your chickpea meringue reaches stiff peaks. Spoon the vegan meringue onto the baking parchment and bake for 1hr 30 mins, or until they come off the paper easily. Leave to cool.
- Meanwhile, mix the berries with the icing sugar and rose water. Set aside for 30 mins so the flavours infuse and the berries release some of their juices.
- Put the yogurt into a large bowl, crush in the meringues then stir through 1/3 of the fruit, rippling it through the yogurt. Spoon into 4 serving dishes then top with the remaining fruit and the rose petals.

Nutrition Information

- Calories: 383 calories
- Fiber: 5 grams fiber
- Sodium: 0.2 milligram of sodium
- Total Carbohydrate: 46 grams carbohydrates
- Sugar: 42 grams sugar
- Total Fat: 19 grams fat
- Saturated Fat: 17 grams saturated fat
- Protein: 4 grams protein

136. Vegan Gingerbread People

Serving: makes around 20 | Prep: 30mins | Cook: 12mins | Ready in:

Ingredients

- 1 tbsp chia seeds
- 400g plain flour, plus extra for dusting
- 200g coconut oil
- 2 tbsp ground ginger
- 1 tsp ground cinnamon
- 200g dark muscovado sugar
- 50g maple syrup
- 100ml aquafaba (water from a can of chickpeas)
- 500g icing sugar
- ½ tsp lemon juice

Direction

- Put the chia seeds in a small bowl and stir in 3 tbsp water. Leave to soak for 5-10 mins until gloopy. Meanwhile put the flour into a large mixing bowl and rub in the coconut oil until it's almost disappeared into the flour. Stir in the spices.
- In another bowl mix together the sugar, maple syrup, chia mixture and 2 tbsp water until smooth then pour over the flour. Stir until well combined then knead together to make a soft dough. Wrap in cling film until ready to use.
- Heat oven to 180C/160C fan/gas 6. Roll out the dough on a lightly floured surface then cut into gingerbread people (or whatever shape you like) and bake for 10-12 mins on baking sheets lined with baking parchment until just starting to darken at the edges. Let them cool for a couple of minutes on the tray then transfer to a wire rack to cool.
- While the gingerbread cools whip the aquafaba in a bowl using electric beaters until really foamy. Add 3/4 of the icing sugar and whisk until smooth and thick, then whisk in the rest of the icing sugar and the lemon juice. Whisk again until the mixture forms stiff

peaks. Transfer to a piping bag until ready to use. Snip a little off the end of the piping bag and use to create designs and faces on your gingerbread.

Nutrition Information

- Calories: 315 calories
- Total Fat: 10 grams fat
- Saturated Fat: 9 grams saturated fat
- Fiber: 1 grams fiber
- Sugar: 36 grams sugar
- Protein: 2 grams protein
- Sodium: 0.01 milligram of sodium
- Total Carbohydrate: 52 grams carbohydrates

137.   Vegan Lemon Cheesecake

Serving: 12 | Prep: 15mins | Cook: | Ready in:

Ingredients

- For the base
- 30g coconut oil, plus extra for greasing
- 100g blanched almonds
- 100g soft pitted dates
- For the topping
- 300g cashew nuts
- 2 ½ tbsp agave syrup
- 50g coconut oil
- 150ml almond milk
- 2 lemons, zested and juiced

Direction

- Put the cashews in a large bowl, pour over boiling water and leave to soak for 1 hr. Meanwhile, blitz the ingredients for the base with a pinch of salt in a food processor. Grease a 23cm tart tin with coconut oil, then press the mix into the base and pop in the fridge to set (about 30 mins).

- Drain the cashews and tip into the cleaned out food processor. Add all the remaining topping ingredients, reserving a quarter of the lemon zest in damp kitchen paper to serve, then blitz until smooth. Spoon onto the base and put in the fridge to set completely (about 2 hrs). Just before serving, scatter over the reserved lemon zest.

Nutrition Information

- Calories: 297 calories
- Sugar: 10 grams sugar
- Fiber: 1 grams fiber
- Total Fat: 22 grams fat
- Saturated Fat: 8 grams saturated fat
- Protein: 7 grams protein
- Sodium: 0.1 milligram of sodium
- Total Carbohydrate: 16 grams carbohydrates

138.   Vegan Millionaire's Bars

Serving: makes 16 | Prep: 30mins | Cook: 5mins | Ready in:

Ingredients

- For the base
- 150g cashew nuts
- 50g rolled oat
- 4 medjool dates, pitted
- 50g coconut oil, melted
- For the filling
- 350g pitted medjool dates
- 125ml unsweetened almond milk
- 25ml maple syrup
- 150g coconut oil
- 1 tsp vanilla extract
- For the topping
- 150g coconut oil
- 5 tbsp cocoa powder
- 2 tsp maple syrup

Direction

- Grease a 20cm square cake tin and line with baking parchment. Tip the cashew nuts and oats into a food processer and blitz to crumbs. Add the dates and coconut oil, and blend again. Transfer to the tin and use a spoon to press the nutty mixture into a compact, even layer that covers the base. Chill while you prepare the filling.
- For the filling, add the dates, almond milk, maple syrup and coconut oil to a saucepan with a generous pinch of salt and bring to a simmer. Boil for 2-3 mins until the dates are really soft, then tip into the blender, add the vanilla extract and blitz to a smooth purée. Add a little more salt if the mixture is too sweet. Pour over the nutty base and spread to the sides of the tin, getting the surface as smooth as possible. Chill while you prepare the topping.
- Gently heat the coconut oil in a saucepan until melted. Remove from the heat and whisk in the cocoa and maple syrup until there are no lumps. Cool for 10 mins, pour over the caramel layer and return to the fridge for at least 3 hrs or until firmly set. To serve, cut into squares. Will keep in the fridge for up to 1 week.

Nutrition Information

- Calories: 373 calories
- Total Carbohydrate: 25 grams carbohydrates
- Sugar: 20 grams sugar
- Fiber: 3 grams fiber
- Protein: 4 grams protein
- Total Fat: 28 grams fat
- Saturated Fat: 20 grams saturated fat

Chapter 7: Dairy-Free Kids' Recipes

***

139.   5 A Day Tagine

Serving: 4 | Prep: 10mins | Cook: 35mins | Ready in:

Ingredients

- 4 carrots, cut into chunks
- 4 small parsnips, or 3 large, cut into chunks
- 3 red onions, cut into wedges
- 2 red peppers, deseeded and cut into chunks
- 2 tbsp olive oil
- 1 tsp each ground cumin, paprika, cinnamon and mild chilli powder
- 400g can chopped tomato
- 2 small handfuls soft dried apricots
- 2 tsp honey

Direction

- Heat oven to 200C/fan 180C/gas 6. Scatter the veg over a couple of baking trays, drizzle with half the oil, season, then rub the oil over the veg with your hands to coat. Roast for 30 mins until tender and beginning to brown.
- Meanwhile, fry the spices in the remaining oil for 1 min – they should sizzle and start to smell aromatic. Tip in the tomatoes, apricots, honey and a can of water. Simmer for 5 mins until the sauce is slightly reduced and the apricots plump, then stir in the veg and some seasoning. Serve with couscous or jacket potatoes.

Nutrition Information

- Calories: 272 calories
- Total Carbohydrate: 45 grams carbohydrates
- Sugar: 32 grams sugar
- Protein: 7 grams protein
- Sodium: 0.35 milligram of sodium
- Total Fat: 8 grams fat
- Saturated Fat: 1 grams saturated fat

140. Bean & Bangers One Pot

Serving: 4 | Prep: 10mins | Cook: 30mins | Ready in:

Ingredients

- 1 tbsp olive oil
- 8 good-quality pork sausages (Toulouse or Sicilian varieties work well)
- 2 carrots, halved lengthways and sliced
- 2 onions, finely chopped
- 2 tbsp red wine vinegar
- 2 x 410g cans mixed beans in water, rinsed and drained
- 400ml chicken stock
- 100g frozen pea
- 2 tbsp Dijon mustard

Direction

- Heat the oil in a large pan. Sizzle the sausages for about 6 mins, turning occasionally, until brown on all sides, then remove to a plate. Tip the carrots and onions into the pan, then cook for 8 mins, stirring occasionally, until the onions are soft. Add the vinegar to the pan, then stir in the drained beans. Pour over the stock, nestle the sausages in with the beans, then simmer everything for 10 mins.
- Scatter in the frozen peas, cook for 2 mins more until heated through, then take off the heat and stir in the mustard. Season to taste. Serve scooped straight from the pan.

Nutrition Information

- Calories: 569 calories
- Total Fat: 31 grams fat
- Saturated Fat: 9 grams saturated fat
- Fiber: 11 grams fiber
- Sugar: 13 grams sugar
- Total Carbohydrate: 41 grams carbohydrates
- Protein: 35 grams protein
- Sodium: 2.81 milligram of sodium

141. Beef & Swede Casserole

Serving: 4 | Prep: 15mins | Cook: 1hours25mins | Ready in:

Ingredients

- 2 tbsp vegetable oil
- 2 onions, sliced
- ½ celery stick, sliced
- 500g diced braising beef
- 200ml red wine (optional)
- 700ml beef stock (or chicken)
- 500g swede, peeled and cut into chunky dice
- 300g floury potatoes (such as Maris Piper), diced
- 3 thyme sprigs
- 1 bay leaf
- green vegetables, to serve (optional)

Direction

- Heat the oil in a flameproof casserole dish over a medium-high heat. Fry the onions and celery for a few mins until turning brown. Add the beef and brown all over for 3-4 mins. Pour in the wine, if using, and let it reduce by half. Add the stock and toss in the swede, potatoes, thyme and bay leaf. Season and bring to the boil.
- Reduce the heat, cover with a lid and leave for 1 hr. If you want to reduce the liquid a little, remove the lid, turn up the heat and cook for a further 10-15 mins or until the sauce has thickened.
- Season to taste and remove the thyme sprigs and bay leaf. Serve with some green veg, if you like.

Nutrition Information

- Calories: 352 calories
- Protein: 30 grams protein
- Sodium: 0.6 milligram of sodium
- Fiber: 5 grams fiber

- Total Carbohydrate: 20 grams carbohydrates
- Total Fat: 15 grams fat
- Saturated Fat: 4 grams saturated fat
- Sugar: 7 grams sugar

142. Butter Bean, Chorizo & Spinach Baked Eggs

Serving: 2 | Prep: 5mins | Cook: 15mins | Ready in:

Ingredients

- ½ tbsp olive oil
- 1 red onion, sliced
- 1 garlic clove, chopped
- 1 tsp chilli flakes
- 100g chorizo, sliced into thin rounds
- 400g can butter beans, drained
- 100g spinach
- 4 medium eggs
- small handful coriander (optional)

Direction

- Heat oven to 220C/200C fan/gas 7. Heat the oil in a medium frying pan (ovenproof if you have one) over a medium heat. Add the onion and cook for 3 mins until starting to soften.
- Add the garlic, chilli flakes and chorizo, and fry for another 2 mins before adding the butter beans and a generous pinch of salt. Stir to combine, then cook for 2 mins more. Add the spinach and a splash of water and stir until wilted. Remove from the heat.
- If your pan isn't ovenproof, tip the mixture into a medium casserole dish. Make four dips in the mixture with the back of a tablespoon and crack the eggs into each hole. Sprinkle with salt and freshly ground pepper (and extra chilli, if you like), then bake for 5-6 mins until the egg whites are set and the yolk is still runny. Serve with a scattering of chopped coriander, if you like.

Nutrition Information

- Calories: 504 calories
- Protein: 34 grams protein
- Total Fat: 29 grams fat
- Sodium: 2.3 milligram of sodium
- Total Carbohydrate: 22 grams carbohydrates
- Sugar: 6 grams sugar
- Fiber: 9 grams fiber
- Saturated Fat: 9 grams saturated fat

143. Butternut Soup With Crispy Sage & Apple Croutons

Serving: 4 | Prep: 20mins | Cook: 30mins | Ready in:

Ingredients

- 1 tbsp olive oil
- 1 large onion, chopped
- 1 garlic clove, chopped
- 1 butternut squash, about 1kg, peeled, deseeded and chopped
- 3 tbsp madeira or dry Sherry
- 500ml gluten-free vegetable stock, plus a little extra if necessary
- 1 tsp chopped sage, plus 20 small leaves, cleaned and dried
- sunflower oil, for frying
- For the apple croutons
- 1 tbsp olive oil
- 1 large eating apple, peeled, cored and diced
- a few pinches of golden caster sugar

Direction

- Heat the oil in a large pan, add the onion and fry for 5 mins. Add the garlic and squash, and cook for 5 mins more. Pour in the Madeira and stock, stir in the chopped sage, then cover and simmer for 20 mins until the squash is tender.
- Blitz with a hand blender or in a food processor until completely smooth. Allow to cool in the pan, then chill until ready to serve. Will keep for 2 days or freeze for 3 months. To

make the crispy sage, heat some oil (a depth of about 2cm) in a small pan, then drop in the sage leaves until they are crisp – you will need to do this in batches. Drain on kitchen paper. Will keep for several hours.

- Just before serving, reheat the soup in a pan. The texture should be quite thick and velvety, but thin it with a little stock if it is too thick.
- For the apple croutons, heat the oil in a large pan, add the apple and fry until starting to soften. Sprinkle with the sugar and stir until lightly caramelised.
- To serve, ladle the soup into small bowls and top with the apple, sage and a grinding of black pepper.

Nutrition Information

- Calories: 231 calories
- Total Fat: 7 grams fat
- Saturated Fat: 1 grams saturated fat
- Protein: 4 grams protein
- Total Carbohydrate: 31 grams carbohydrates
- Sodium: 0.4 milligram of sodium
- Sugar: 20 grams sugar
- Fiber: 8 grams fiber

144.	Cherry Tomato, Thyme & Bacon Flan

Serving: 8 | Prep: 35mins | Cook: 45mins | Ready in:

Ingredients

- 50g wholemeal flour
- 85g vegetable baking margarine
- 100g plain flour
- 1 large egg, beaten
- 150g natural Yofu (a 100% dairy-free yogurt)
- 1 small onion, diced
- 1 tbsp vegetable oil
- 4 tbsp soya milk
- leaves from 2 sprigs thyme, plus a few extra sprigs

- 150g cherry tomato, halved
- 2 thick-cut rashers unsmoked bacon, chopped

Direction

- Preheat the oven to 220C/gas 7/ fan 200C. Put the flours in a bowl and rub in the margarine until it resembles breadcrumbs. Mix in 4-5 tsp water to make a soft dough. Turn on to a lightly floured surface, roll out and use to line a 20cm flan tin. Line with baking parchment, cover with baking beans and bake for 5 minutes. Remove the paper and beans and bake for 5 minutes more. Allow to cool on a rack. Reduce the oven to 160C/gas 3/fan oven 140C.
- Heat the oil in a pan and cook the bacon and onion until crispy. Remove from the heat.
- Mix the soya milk, Yofu, eggs and thyme leaves. Season well. Put the onion, bacon and tomatoes in the flan case. Add the milk mixture and top with extra thyme sprigs on top. Bake for 30 minutes until set.

Nutrition Information

- Calories: 302 calories
- Protein: 9 grams protein
- Sodium: 0.49 milligram of sodium
- Total Fat: 21 grams fat
- Saturated Fat: 4 grams saturated fat
- Total Carbohydrate: 21 grams carbohydrates
- Fiber: 2 grams fiber

145.	Chicken, Sweet Potato & Coconut Curry

Serving: Serves 2 adults and 2 children | Prep: | Cook: | Ready in:

Ingredients

- 1 tbsp sunflower oil
- 2 tsp mild curry paste

- 2 large boneless, skinless chicken breasts, cut into bite-size pieces
- 2 medium-sized sweet potatoes, peeled and cut into bite-size pieces
- 4 tbsp red split lentils
- 300ml chicken stock
- 400ml can coconut milk
- 175g frozen peas

Direction

- Heat the oil in a deep frying pan or wok, stir in the curry paste and fry for 1 minute. Add the chicken, sweet potatoes and lentils and stir to coat in the paste, then pour in the stock and coconut milk. Bring to the boil, then simmer for 15 minutes.
- Tip in the peas, bring back to the boil and simmer for a further 4-5 minutes. Season to taste before serving.

Nutrition Information

- Calories: 291 calories
- Sodium: 0.57 milligram of sodium
- Total Fat: 14 grams fat
- Saturated Fat: 10 grams saturated fat
- Total Carbohydrate: 24.5 grams carbohydrates
- Fiber: 3.6 grams fiber
- Protein: 19 grams protein

146. Easy Chicken Gumbo

Serving: 4 | Prep: 15mins | Cook: 40mins | Ready in:

Ingredients

- 2 tbsp olive oil
- 200g smoked bacon lardons
- 1 onion, sliced
- 130g pack Padrón peppers, stalks removed, sliced (or 1 green chilli and 100g green pepper)
- 4 skinless chicken breasts, cut into bite-sized pieces

- 3 tbsp plain flour
- 1 tbsp Cajun spice mix
- 3 garlic cloves, crushed
- 500ml chicken stock
- 175g pack okra, sliced (or 2 courgettes, sliced)
- 500g carton passata
- 2 spring onions, sliced
- cooked rice and black beans, to serve

Direction

- Heat the oil in a large pan, add the lardons and onion, and fry for 5 mins until the bacon is starting to crisp and the onion is soft. Add the peppers, chicken and flour, and fry for a further 5 mins or until the chicken is golden brown and the flour is starting to take on a a a biscuty colour.
- Stir in the Cajun spice mix and garlic, then slowly add the chicken stock, stirring all the time. Add the okra, passata and some seasoning and simmer for 20 mins, uncovered, over a medium heat. Stir frequently during cooking to loosen the flour from the base of the pan.
- Sprinkle over the spring onions and serve with rice and black beans.

Nutrition Information

- Calories: 489 calories
- Fiber: 6 grams fiber
- Sugar: 9 grams sugar
- Saturated Fat: 7 grams saturated fat
- Total Fat: 22 grams fat
- Sodium: 2.1 milligram of sodium
- Total Carbohydrate: 22 grams carbohydrates
- Protein: 48 grams protein

147. Favourite Pasta Salad

Serving: Makes 4 portions | Prep: 10mins | Cook: 12mins | Ready in:

Ingredients

- 250g pasta shapes (use vegan-friendly dried pasta)
- 140g frozen peas
- pack parsley, chopped
- small pack chives, snipped
- zest and juice 1 lemon
- 2 tbsp olive oil

Direction

- Cook the pasta, adding the peas for final 2 mins cooking time. Drain, rinse with cold water to cool, then drain again. Tip into a bowl with the chopped herbs, lemon zest and juice, olive oil and plenty of seasoning and mix well. Cover and chill, spooning out portions as and when. If you're making this for one person, by days 3 and 4 you'll need to stir in a little olive oil or something creamy to loosen the pasta.

Nutrition Information

- Calories: 292 calories
- Total Carbohydrate: 51 grams carbohydrates
- Sugar: 3 grams sugar
- Total Fat: 7 grams fat
- Protein: 10 grams protein
- Sodium: 0.02 milligram of sodium
- Saturated Fat: 1 grams saturated fat
- Fiber: 4 grams fiber

148.   Lemon & Rosemary Crusted Fish Fillets

Serving: 4 | Prep: 10mins | Cook: 8mins |Ready in:

Ingredients

- 4 white fish fillets (hake is sustainable)
- 2 rosemary sprigs, leaves chopped, or 1 tsp dried
- 50g bread (about 2 slices), torn into pieces
- zest 2 lemons, plus wedges to serve
- 1 tbsp olive oil

Direction

- Heat the grill to medium. Place the fish fillets, skin-side up, on a baking tray, then grill for 4 mins. Meanwhile, place the rosemary, bread, lemon zest and some seasoning in a food processor, then blitz to make fine crumbs.
- Turn the fish over, then press a quarter of the crumbs over the top of each fillet. Drizzle with olive oil, then grill for 4 mins until the crust is golden and the fish is cooked through and just flaking. Serve with buttered new potatoes and lemon wedges for squeezing over.

Nutrition Information

- Calories: 184 calories
- Total Fat: 6 grams fat
- Saturated Fat: 1 grams saturated fat
- Total Carbohydrate: 6 grams carbohydrates
- Protein: 26 grams protein
- Sodium: 0.51 milligram of sodium

149.   Lentil Lasagne

Serving: 4 | Prep: 15mins | Cook: 1hours15mins |Ready in:

Ingredients

- 1 tbsp olive oil
- 1 onion, chopped
- 1 carrot, chopped
- 1 celery stick, chopped
- 1 garlic clove, crushed
- 2 x 400g cans lentils, drained, rinsed
- 1 tbsp cornflour
- 400g can chopped tomato
- 1 tsp mushroom ketchup
- 1 tsp chopped oregano (or 1 tsp dried)
- 1 tsp vegetable stock powder

- 2 cauliflower heads, broken into florets
- 2 tbsp unsweetened soya milk
- pinch of freshly grated nutmeg
- 9 dried egg-free lasagne sheets

Direction

- Heat the oil in a pan, add the onion, carrot and celery, and gently cook for 10-15 mins until soft. Add the garlic, cook for a few mins, then stir in the lentils and cornflour.
- Add the tomatoes plus a canful of water, the mushroom ketchup, oregano, stock powder and some seasoning. Simmer for 15 mins, stirring occasionally.
- Meanwhile, cook the cauliflower in a pan of boiling water for 10 mins or until tender. Drain, then purée with the soya milk using a hand blender or food processor. Season well and add the nutmeg.
- Heat oven to 180C/160C fan/gas 4. Spread a third of the lentil mixture over the base of a ceramic baking dish, about 20 x 30cm. Cover with a single layer of lasagne, snapping the sheets to fit. Add another third of the lentil mixture, then spread a third of the cauliflower purée on top, followed by a layer of pasta. Top with the last third of lentils and lasagna, followed by the remaining purée.
- Cover loosely with foil and bake for 35-45 mins, removing the foil for the final 10 mins of cooking.

Nutrition Information

- Calories: 378 calories
- Total Carbohydrate: 63 grams carbohydrates
- Sodium: 0.3 milligram of sodium
- Total Fat: 6 grams fat
- Saturated Fat: 1 grams saturated fat
- Sugar: 11 grams sugar
- Protein: 19 grams protein
- Fiber: 10 grams fiber

150. Minty Pea & Potato Soup

Serving: 4 | Prep: 5mins | Cook: 25mins | Ready in:

Ingredients

- 2 tsp vegetable oil
- 1 onion, chopped
- 800g potato, peeled and cut into small chunks
- vegetable stock
- 350g frozen pea
- handful mint, chopped

Direction

- Heat the oil in a large saucepan, then fry the onion for 5 mins until softened. Add the potatoes and stock, then bring to the boil. Cover and simmer for 10-15 mins until tender, adding the peas 2 mins before the end of the cooking time.
- Use a slotted spoon to remove a quarter of the vegetables from the pan and set aside. Blend the remaining vegetables and stock in a food processor or using a hand blender until smooth, then stir through the reserved veg, chopped mint and some seasoning. Serve with bread on the side.

Nutrition Information

- Calories: 249 calories
- Total Fat: 3 grams fat
- Saturated Fat: 1 grams saturated fat
- Total Carbohydrate: 48 grams carbohydrates
- Sugar: 7 grams sugar
- Protein: 11 grams protein
- Sodium: 0.36 milligram of sodium

151. Oven Baked Thai Chicken Rice

Serving: 4 | Prep: | Cook: 30mins | Ready in:

Ingredients

- 1 tbsp vegetable oil
- 1 onion, chopped
- 400g pack mini chicken fillet
- 4 tbsp Thai green curry paste (we used Bart's), or use less for a milder taste
- 250g basmati and wild rice mix, rinsed (we used Tilda)
- 2 red peppers, deseeded and cut into wedges
- finely grated zest and juice 1 lime
- 400g reduced-fat coconut milk
- handful coriander leaves, to serve

Direction

- Heat oven to 200C/fan 180C/gas 6. Heat the oil in a shallow ovenproof casserole dish, then soften the onion for 5 mins. Add the chicken and curry paste, then cook for 3 mins, stirring to coat.
- Tip in the rice and peppers, then stir in the lime zest and juice, coconut milk and 250ml boiling water. Bring to the boil, then pop the lid on and bake for 20 mins until the rice is fluffy. Scatter with coriander before serving.

Nutrition Information

- Calories: 510 calories
- Total Fat: 18 grams fat
- Protein: 32 grams protein
- Saturated Fat: 10 grams saturated fat
- Total Carbohydrate: 59 grams carbohydrates
- Sugar: 6 grams sugar
- Sodium: 1.02 milligram of sodium
- Fiber: 2 grams fiber

152.   Peanut Butter Chicken

Serving: 4 | Prep: 10mins | Cook: 40mins | Ready in:

Ingredients

- 2 tbsp vegetable oil

- 8 skinless boneless chicken thighs, cut into chunks
- 1 garlic clove, crushed
- 2 red chillies, finely sliced (deseeded if you don't like it too hot)
- 2 tsp fresh ginger, grated
- 2 tsp garam masala
- 100g smooth peanut butter
- 400ml can coconut milk
- 400g can chopped tomatoes
- 1 small bunch coriander, ½ roughly chopped, ½ leaves picked
- roasted peanuts, to serve
- cooked basmati rice, to serve

Direction

- Heat 1 tbsp of the oil in a deep frying pan over a medium heat. Brown the chicken in batches, setting aside once golden. Fry the garlic, chilli and ginger in the other 1 tbsp oil for 1 min. Add the garam masala and fry for 1 min more.
- Stir in the peanut butter, coconut milk and tomatoes, and bring to a simmer. Return the chicken to the pan and add the chopped coriander. Cook for 30 mins until the sauce thickens and the chicken is cooked through.
- Serve with the remaining coriander, roasted peanuts and rice, if you like.

Nutrition Information

- Calories: 572 calories
- Protein: 33 grams protein
- Total Fat: 43 grams fat
- Sugar: 7 grams sugar
- Sodium: 0.3 milligram of sodium
- Total Carbohydrate: 11 grams carbohydrates
- Fiber: 3 grams fiber
- Saturated Fat: 20 grams saturated fat

153. Pepper & Walnut Hummus With Veggie Dippers

Serving: 2 | Prep: 10mins | Cook: 6mins | Ready in:

Ingredients

- 400g can chickpeas, drained
- 1 garlic clove
- 1 large roasted red pepper from a jar (not in oil), about 100g
- 1 tbsp tahini paste
- juice ½ lemon
- 4 walnut halves, chopped
- 2 courgettes, cut into batons
- 2 carrots, cut into batons
- 2 celery sticks, cut into batons

Direction

- Put the chickpeas, garlic, pepper, tahini and lemon juice in a bowl. Blitz with a hand blender or in a food processor to make a thick purée. Stir in the walnuts. Pack into pots, if you like, and serve with the veggie sticks. Will keep in the fridge for two days, although the vegetables are best prepared fresh to preserve their vitamins.

Nutrition Information

- Calories: 296 calories
- Sodium: 0.8 milligram of sodium
- Protein: 14 grams protein
- Total Carbohydrate: 30 grams carbohydrates
- Sugar: 9 grams sugar
- Fiber: 12 grams fiber
- Total Fat: 14 grams fat
- Saturated Fat: 2 grams saturated fat

154. Salmon & Lemon Mini Fish Cakes

Serving: Makes 20 | Prep: 30mins | Cook: 15mins | Ready in:

Ingredients

- 2 large baking potatoes
- 2 tbsp olive oil
- grated zest and juice ½ lemon
- 1 egg yolk
- 140g smoked salmon trimmings, plus extra to serve
- 1 tbsp chopped parsley, plust extra
- 2 tbsp gluten-free flour mixed with 1 tsp coarsely ground pepper
- a little oil, for frying

Direction

- Microwave potatoes on high for 10 mins until tender. Leave to cool for 5 mins, scoop the flesh in a bowl, then mash and leave to cool. Season with olive oil, lemon zest and juice to taste, then mix in the egg, salmon and parsley. Shape into small rounds 3cm wide and 1cm deep. Chill for 15 mins.
- Dust each cake with the peppered flour, then fry over a low heat in a little oil for 2-3 mins on each side. Drain on kitchen paper and serve garnished with salmon and parsley.

Nutrition Information

- Calories: 52 calories
- Saturated Fat: 1 grams saturated fat
- Total Carbohydrate: 3 grams carbohydrates
- Protein: 2 grams protein
- Sodium: 0.34 milligram of sodium
- Total Fat: 4 grams fat

155. Spanish Chicken Pie

Serving: 4 | Prep: 10mins | Cook: 30mins | Ready in:

Ingredients

- 1kg potatoes, chopped
- 3 tsp paprika (use smoked paprika if you have it)
- 2 tsp olive oil
- 2 onions, sliced
- 2 garlic cloves, crushed
- 2 x 400g cans chopped tomatoes
- 300g cooked chicken, shredded
- 140g roasted pepper from a jar, sliced (we like Karyatis)
- handful Kalamata olives, halved

Direction

- Heat oven to 200C/fan 180C/gas 6. Boil the potatoes for 15-20 mins until tender. Drain, return to the pan, then mash with some seasoning and 2 tsp of the paprika.
- Meanwhile, heat the oil in a large pan, then fry the onions and garlic for a few mins until softened. Stir in the remaining paprika for 1 min, add the tomatoes , then, bring to a simmer. Tip into a large ovenproof dish, then stir in the chicken, peppers, olives and some seasoning.
- Spoon over the mash, then bake for 15 mins until the mash is golden on top and the sauce is bubbling.

Nutrition Information

- Calories: 421 calories
- Sugar: 10 grams sugar
- Protein: 30 grams protein
- Saturated Fat: 2 grams saturated fat
- Sodium: 1.32 milligram of sodium
- Fiber: 8 grams fiber
- Total Fat: 10 grams fat
- Total Carbohydrate: 57 grams carbohydrates

156. Sticky Chicken Drumsticks & Sesame Rice Salad

Serving: 2 | Prep: 10mins | Cook: 30mins | Ready in:

Ingredients

- 4 chicken drumsticks
- 2 tbsp clear honey, plus 1tsp
- 2 tbsp tamari (or soy sauce if not gluten free)
- 3 tbsp vegetable oil
- 2 tbsp sesame oil
- 120g basmati rice
- 70g kale, chopped
- juice 2 limes
- 100g radishes, halved
- 1 tbsp sesame seeds

Direction

- Heat oven to 200C/180C fan/gas 6. Put the drumsticks in a roasting tin. Mix 2 tbsp honey, the tamari, 1 tbsp veg oil and 1 tbsp sesame oil in a bowl, then pour over the chicken – make sure each piece is covered. Roast for 25-30 mins.
- Meanwhile, cover the rice with 240ml water and bring to the boil. Cook for 8-10 mins until tender. Massage the kale with 1 tbsp veg oil for 5 mins until softening (this makes it less chewy). Drizzle over the lime juice, remaining sesame oil and honey, and season. Add the radishes and set aside.
- Fry the rice in the remaining veg oil in a non-stick pan to dry out. Add to the kale, and toss to combine.
- Serve the drumsticks with the salad and scatter over the sesame seeds.

Nutrition Information

- Calories: 779 calories
- Total Fat: 39 grams fat
- Fiber: 2 grams fiber

- Sodium: 2.5 milligram of sodium
- Sugar: 20 grams sugar
- Saturated Fat: 6 grams saturated fat
- Protein: 34 grams protein
- Total Carbohydrate: 72 grams carbohydrates

157. Sweet Potato Curly Fries With Barbecue Seasoning

Serving: 4 | Prep: 20mins | Cook: 25mins | Ready in:

Ingredients

- For the curly fries
- 400g sweet potatoes, peeled
- 2 tbsp olive oil
- For the barbecue seasoning
- 1 tsp black onion seeds
- 1 tsp smoked paprika
- ½ tsp ground cumin
- ½ tsp mustard powder
- ¼ tsp celery salt
- ¼ tsp chilli powder
- ½ tsp demerara sugar

Direction

- Heat oven to 200C/180C fan/gas 6. Put the sweet potato through your spiralizer using the large noodle attachment. Lay the noodles out on a large baking tray and drizzle with the olive oil, toss well to coat the noodles making sure they end up as a single layer.
- Bake in the oven for 20-25 mins, tossing around in the tray half way through cooking, until tender and starting to crisp up and char at the edges.
- While the fries are baking mix all of the seasoning ingredients together in a bowl and add 1/4 tsp black pepper and 1/4 tsp salt. Stir well and set aside.
- When the fries are ready evenly scatter over the seasoning while they are still hot then transfer to a serving dish.

Nutrition Information

- Calories: 185 calories
- Saturated Fat: 1 grams saturated fat
- Fiber: 4 grams fiber
- Protein: 2 grams protein
- Sodium: 0.8 milligram of sodium
- Total Carbohydrate: 27 grams carbohydrates
- Total Fat: 6 grams fat
- Sugar: 14 grams sugar

158. Thai Turkey Stir Fry

Serving: 4 | Prep: 10mins | Cook: 15mins | Ready in:

Ingredients

- 300g rice noodles
- 1 tsp sunflower oil
- 400g turkey breast steak, cut into thin strips and any fat removed
- 340g green beans, trimmed and halved
- 1 red onion, sliced
- 2 garlic cloves, sliced
- juice 1 lime, plus extra wedges for serving
- 1 tsp chilli powder
- 1 red chilli, finely chopped
- 1 tbsp fish sauce
- handful mint, roughly chopped
- handful coriander, roughly chopped

Direction

- Cook the rice noodles following pack instructions. Heat the oil in a non-stick pan and fry the turkey over a high heat for 2 mins. Add the beans, onion and garlic, and cook for a further 5 mins.
- Stir in the lime juice, chilli powder, fresh chilli and fish sauce, then cook for 3 mins more. Stir in the noodles and herbs, then toss everything together before serving.

Nutrition Information

- Calories: 425 calories
- Total Carbohydrate: 71 grams carbohydrates
- Sodium: 0.92 milligram of sodium
- Total Fat: 3 grams fat
- Saturated Fat: 1 grams saturated fat
- Sugar: 4 grams sugar
- Fiber: 4 grams fiber
- Protein: 32 grams protein

159.   Tofu Brekkie Pancakes

Serving: 6 | Prep: 10mins | Cook: 10mins | Ready in:

Ingredients

- 50g Brazil nuts
- 3 sliced bananas
- 240g raspberries
- maple syrup or honey, to serve
- For the batter
- 349g pack firm silken tofu
- 2 tsp vanilla extract
- 2 tsp lemon juice
- 400ml unsweetened almond milk
- 1 tbsp vegetable oil, plus 1-2 tbsp extra for frying
- 250g buckwheat flour
- 4 tbsp light muscovado sugar
- 1 ½ tsp ground mixed spice
- 1 tbsp gluten-free baking powder

Direction

- Heat oven to 180C/160C fan/gas 4. Scatter the nuts over a baking tray and cook for 5 mins until toasty and golden. Leave to cool, then chop. Turn the oven down low if you want to keep the whole batch of pancakes warm, although I think they are best enjoyed straight from the pan.
- Put the tofu, vanilla, lemon juice and 200ml of the milk into a deep jug or bowl. Using a stick blender, blend together until liquid, then keep going until it turns thick and smooth, like

yogurt. Stir in the oil and the rest of the milk to loosen the mixture.

- Put the dry ingredients and 1 tsp salt in a large bowl and whisk to combine and aerate. If there are any lumps in the sugar, squish them with your fingers. Make a well in the centre, pour in the tofu mix and bring together to make a thick batter.
- Heat a large (ideally non-stick) frying pan and swirl around 1 tsp oil. For golden pancakes that don't stick, the pan and oil should be hot enough to get an enthusiastic sizzle on contact with the batter, but not so hot that it scorches it. Test a drop.
- Using a ladle or large serving spoon, drop in 3 spoonfuls of batter, easing it out gently in the pan to make pancakes that are about 12cm across. Cook for 2 mins on the first side or until bubbles pop over most of the surface. Loosen with a palette knife, then flip over the pancakes and cook for 1 min more or until puffed up and firm. Transfer to the oven to keep warm, if you need to, but don't stack the pancakes too closely. Cook the rest of the batter, using a little more oil each time. Serve warm with sliced banana, berries, toasted nuts and a good drizzle of maple syrup or honey.

Nutrition Information

- Calories: 377 calories
- Saturated Fat: 2 grams saturated fat
- Fiber: 7 grams fiber
- Sodium: 1.6 milligram of sodium
- Total Fat: 14 grams fat
- Sugar: 21 grams sugar
- Total Carbohydrate: 47 grams carbohydrates
- Protein: 12 grams protein

160.   Vegan Banana Bread

Serving: 10 | Prep: 10mins | Cook: 40mins | Ready in:

Ingredients

- 3 large black bananas
- 75ml vegetable oil or sunflower oil, plus extra for the tin
- 100g brown sugar
- 225g plain flour (or use self-raising flour and reduce the baking powder to 2 heaped tsp)
- 3 heaped tsp baking powder
- 3 tsp cinnamon or mixed spice
- 50g dried fruit or nuts (optional)

Direction

- Heat oven to 200C/180C fan/gas 6. Mash 3 large black peeled bananas with a fork, then mix well with 75g vegetable or sunflower oil and 100g brown sugar.
- Add 225g plain flour, 3 heaped tsp baking powder and 3 tsp cinnamon or mixed spice, and combine well. Add 50g dried fruit or nuts, if using.
- Bake in an oiled, lined 2lb loaf tin for 20 minutes. Check and cover with foil if the cake is browning.
- Bake for another 20 minutes, or until a skewer comes out clean.
- Allow to cool a little before slicing. It's delicious freshly baked, but develops a lovely gooey quality the day after.

Nutrition Information

- Calories: 218 calories
- Sugar: 15 grams sugar
- Protein: 3 grams protein
- Saturated Fat: 1 grams saturated fat
- Total Carbohydrate: 33 grams carbohydrates
- Fiber: 2 grams fiber
- Sodium: 0.5 milligram of sodium
- Total Fat: 8 grams fat

161.   Vegan Brownies

Serving: Makes 12 | Prep: 15mins | Cook: 40mins |Ready in:

Ingredients

- 2 tbsp ground flaxseed
- 200g dark chocolate, roughly chopped
- ½ tsp coffee granules
- 80g vegan margarine, plus extra for greasing
- 125g self-raising flour
- 70g ground almonds
- 50g cocoa powder
- ¼ tsp baking powder
- 250g golden caster sugar
- 1½ tsp vanilla extract

Direction

- Heat oven to 170C/150C fan/gas 3½. Grease and line a 20cm square tin with baking parchment. Combine the flaxseed with 6 tbsp water and set aside for at least 5 mins.
- In a saucepan, melt 120g chocolate, the coffee and margarine with 60ml water on a low heat. Allow to cool slightly.
- Put the flour, almonds, cocoa, baking powder and ¼ tsp salt in a bowl and stir to remove any lumps. Using a hand whisk, mix the sugar into the melted chocolate mixture, and beat well until smooth and glossy, ensuring all the sugar is well dissolved. Stir in the flaxseed mixture, vanilla extract and remaining chocolate, then the flour mixture. Spoon into the prepared tin.
- Bake for 35-45 mins until a skewer inserted in the middle comes out clean with moist crumbs. Allow to cool in the tin completely, then cut into squares. Store in an airtight container and eat within three days.

Nutrition Information

- Calories: 314 calories
- Protein: 5 grams protein
- Sugar: 25 grams sugar
- Total Fat: 16 grams fat
- Saturated Fat: 6 grams saturated fat
- Total Carbohydrate: 36 grams carbohydrates
- Sodium: 0.3 milligram of sodium
- Fiber: 3 grams fiber

162. Vegan Chocolate Banana Ice Cream

Serving: 1 | Prep: 5mins | Cook: |Ready in:

Ingredients

- 1 frozen banana
- 1 tsp cocoa powder

Direction

- In a blender, blitz the frozen banana with the cocoa powder until smooth. Eat straight away.

Nutrition Information

- Calories: 110 calories
- Total Fat: 1 grams fat
- Total Carbohydrate: 23 grams carbohydrates
- Sugar: 21 grams sugar
- Fiber: 2 grams fiber
- Protein: 2 grams protein

Chapter 8: Awesome Dairy-Free Recipes

***

163. Baked Sea Bass With Lemon Caper Dressing

Serving: 4 | Prep: 10mins | Cook: 10mins |Ready in:

Ingredients

- 4 x 100g/4oz sea bass fillets
- olive oil, for brushing

- For the caper dressing
- 3 tbsp extra virgin olive oil
- grated zest 1 lemon, plus 2 tbsp juice
- 2 tbsp small capers
- 2 tsp gluten-free Dijon mustard
- 2 tbsp chopped flat-leaf parsley, plus a few extra leaves (optional)

Direction

- To make the dressing, mix the oil with the lemon zest and juice, capers, mustard, some seasoning and 1 tbsp water. Don't add the parsley yet (unless serving straight away) as the acid in the lemon will fade the colour if they are left together for too long.
- Heat the oven to 220C/200C fan/gas 7. Line a baking tray with baking parchment and put the fish, skin-side up, on top. Brush the skin with oil and sprinkle with some flaky salt. Bake for 7 mins or until the flesh flakes when tested with a knife. Arrange the fish on warm serving plates, spoon over the dressing and scatter with extra parsley leaves, if you like.

Nutrition Information

- Calories: 196 calories
- Total Fat: 13 grams fat
- Saturated Fat: 2 grams saturated fat
- Total Carbohydrate: 1 grams carbohydrates
- Sugar: 1 grams sugar
- Protein: 20 grams protein
- Sodium: 0.8 milligram of sodium

164. Brazilian Prawn & Coconut Stew

Serving: 4 | Prep: 20mins | Cook: 25mins |Ready in:

Ingredients

- 300g long-grain rice
- 1 tbsp vegetable oil

- 1 onion, finely chopped
- 2 garlic cloves, finely chopped
- 1-2 red chillies (deseeded if you don't like it too hot), finely chopped
- 200ml coconut milk
- 400g tomatoes, diced
- 200g green beans, topped and sliced in half
- 300g peeled raw king prawns
- juice 1 lime
- small pack coriander, chopped
- 50g roasted unsalted peanuts, roughly chopped

Direction

- Bring a pan of water to boil and cook the rice following pack instructions.
- Meanwhile, heat the oil in a large frying pan, add the onion, garlic and chillies, and cook for 10 mins on a low heat until soft. Add the coconut milk and bubble for another 4 mins.
- Add the tomatoes and beans, and cook for 5 mins until the tomatoes start to collapse. Add the prawns and cook for 3 mins until pink and cooked through.
- Stir in the lime juice, sprinkle over the coriander and nuts, and serve with the rice.

Nutrition Information

- Calories: 563 calories
- Sugar: 8 grams sugar
- Fiber: 5 grams fiber
- Sodium: 0.4 milligram of sodium
- Total Carbohydrate: 70 grams carbohydrates
- Protein: 25 grams protein
- Total Fat: 19 grams fat
- Saturated Fat: 9 grams saturated fat

---

165.   Butter Bean & Tomato Salad

Serving: 8 | Prep: | Cook: | Ready in:

Ingredients

- 420g can butter beans, drained and rinsed
- 500g cherry tomato, quartered
- 2small green or yellow courgettes (about 300g/10oz in total), chopped into small dice
- 1small red onion, chopped
- 15-20g pack fresh coriander, chopped
- 2 tbsp lemon juice
- 3 tbsp olive oil
- 1 tsp ground cumin

Direction

- Tip all the ingredients into a bowl with some salt and pepper and mix well. Cover and leave at room temperature until ready to serve. This salad can happily be made the day before and chilled.
- On the day, bring the salad to room temperature and give it a good stir before serving.

Nutrition Information

- Calories: 109 calories
- Total Carbohydrate: 9 grams carbohydrates
- Fiber: 3 grams fiber
- Protein: 4 grams protein
- Sodium: 0.41 milligram of sodium
- Total Fat: 6 grams fat
- Saturated Fat: 1 grams saturated fat

---

166.   Coconut & Banana Pancakes

Serving: 10 | Prep: 10mins | Cook: 15mins | Ready in:

Ingredients

- 150g plain flour
- 2 tsp baking powder
- 3 tbsp golden caster sugar
- 400ml can coconut milk, shaken well

- vegetable oil, for frying
- 1-2 bananas, thinly sliced
- 2 passion fruits, flesh scooped out

Direction

- Sift the flour and baking powder into a bowl, and stir in 2 tbsp of the sugar and a pinch of salt. Pour the coconut milk into a bowl, whisk to mix in any fat that has separated, then measure out 300ml into a jug. Stir the milk slowly into the flour mixture to make a smooth batter, or whizz everything in a blender.
- Heat a shallow frying pan or flat griddle and brush it with oil. Use 2 tbsp of batter to make each pancake, frying two at a time – any more will make it difficult to flip them. Push 4-5 pieces of banana into each pancake and cook until bubbles start to pop on the surface, and the edges look dry. They will be a little more delicate than egg-based pancakes, so turn them over carefully and cook the other sides for 1 min. Repeat to make 8-10 pancakes.
- Meanwhile, put the remaining coconut milk and sugar in a small pan. Add a pinch of salt and simmer until the mixture thickens to the consistency of single cream. Use this as a sauce for the pancakes and spoon over some of the passion fruit seeds.

Nutrition Information

- Calories: 179 calories
- Sodium: 0.2 milligram of sodium
- Total Carbohydrate: 23 grams carbohydrates
- Protein: 2 grams protein
- Total Fat: 8 grams fat
- Saturated Fat: 6 grams saturated fat
- Sugar: 11 grams sugar
- Fiber: 1 grams fiber

| 167. | Dairy Free Pancakes |

Serving: Makes 8 small pancakes | Prep: 5mins | Cook: 25mins | Ready in:

Ingredients

- 125g plain flour
- 1 egg
- 300ml hemp or coconut milk (see tip)
- sunflower or rice bran oil, for frying

Direction

- Put the flour in a bowl and make a well in the centre. Crack the egg in the middle and pour in a quarter of the milk. Use an electric or balloon whisk to thoroughly combine the mixture. Once you have a paste, mix in another quarter and once lump free, mix in the remaining milk. Leave to rest for 20 mins. Stir again before using.
- Heat a small, non-stick frying pan with a splash of oil. When hot, pour a small amount of the mixture into the pan and swirl around to coat the base – you want a thin layer. Cook for a few mins until golden brown on the bottom, then turn over and cook until golden on the other side. Repeat until you have used all the mixture, stirring the mixture in between pancakes and adding more oil for frying as necessary. Pile the pancakes up between sheets of baking parchment or cook to order. Serve with the pancake filling of choice.

Nutrition Information

- Calories: 90 calories
- Total Fat: 3.2 grams fat
- Saturated Fat: 0.5 grams saturated fat
- Total Carbohydrate: 12.6 grams carbohydrates
- Sugar: 0.8 grams sugar
- Fiber: 0.7 grams fiber
- Protein: 2.3 grams protein

168. Dosa

Serving: Makes 8-10 | Prep: 10mins | Cook: 10mins | Ready in:

Ingredients

- 50g split urad lentils, washed
- 1 tbsp channa dal /bengal gram
- 190g basmati rice
- 1 tbsp fenugreek seeds (optional)
- vegetable oil, for frying

Direction

- Wash all the ingredients, except for the oil, three or four times, then drain. Leave to soak in cold water in a bowl overnight.
- Drain the water from the ingredients, but keep it and set aside. Transfer the soaked ingredients to a food processor and grind to make a smooth paste. Make sure the batter doesn't look grainy – you can use a little of the soaking water if you need to. It should be like a thick, smooth pancake batter and should coat the back of a spoon. Empty into a large bowl and cover. Keep it in a warm place overnight to allow the batter to ferment (see tip, below). It will have doubled in quantity and look bubbly. If you're not using the batter straight away, chill for later. It will keep for up to five days.
- Very gently stir the batter. It will have thickened in consistency, so you can add a little water to give it a thick but pourable consistency.
- Heat a non-stick frying pan on a low to medium heat for 5 mins. Drizzle over a few drops of oil, then wipe the pan with kitchen paper to get rid of any excess oil.
- Sprinkle a handful of water on the hot pan to cool it, then dry with some kitchen paper. Pour one ladle of the dosa batter in the middle of the pan. Using the bottom of the ladle, quickly move it in a circular motion, allowing the batter to spread outwards from the middle towards the edge of the pan, to form a round, thin pancake.

- Drizzle a few drops of oil all over the dosa and increase the temperature to a high heat. When it turns slightly golden and the edges begin to lift, add any stuffing (like dosa masala potato stuffing) to the middle. Continue to cook until the underside looks completely golden and crisp. Use a flat spatula to loosen the edges, then roll over the potato stuffing and lift onto a plate.
- Before you make the next dosa, decrease the temperature of the pan back to a medium heat and repeat the above steps.

Nutrition Information

- Calories: 94 calories
- Sodium: 0.01 milligram of sodium
- Saturated Fat: 0.2 grams saturated fat
- Fiber: 1 grams fiber
- Protein: 3 grams protein
- Total Carbohydrate: 16 grams carbohydrates
- Sugar: 0.2 grams sugar
- Total Fat: 2 grams fat

169. Easy Vegan Pancakes

Serving: Serves 4-6 (makes 16 pancakes) | Prep: 5mins | Cook: 30mins | Ready in:

Ingredients

- 300g self-raising flour
- 1 tsp baking powder
- 1 tbsp sugar (any kind)
- 1 tbsp vanilla extract
- 400ml plant-based milk (such as oat, almond or soya)
- 1 tbsp vegetable oil for cooking
- To serve (optional)
- banana slices, blueberries, maple syrup, vegan chocolate chips, plant-based yogurt

Direction

- Whisk the flour, baking powder, sugar, vanilla extract and a pinch of salt in a bowl using a balloon whisk until mixed. Slowly pour in the milk until you get a smooth, thick batter.
- Heat a little of the oil in a non-stick frying pan over a medium-low heat, and add 2 tbsp batter into the pan at a time to make small, round pancakes. You will need to do this in batches of two-three at a time. Cook for 3-4 mins until the edges are set, and bubbles are appearing on the surface. Flip the pancakes over and cook for another 2-3 mins until golden on both sides and cooked through. Keep warm in a low oven while you cook the remaining pancakes.
- Serve stacked with lots of toppings of your choice, or serve with bowls of toppings for everyone to help themselves.

Nutrition Information

- Calories: 90 calories
- Sodium: 0.23 milligram of sodium
- Total Carbohydrate: 16 grams carbohydrates
- Total Fat: 1 grams fat
- Sugar: 2 grams sugar
- Fiber: 1 grams fiber
- Saturated Fat: 0.2 grams saturated fat
- Protein: 3 grams protein

170.   Hot BBQ Beef, Horseradish & Pasta Salad

Serving: 4 | Prep: | Cook: 15mins | Ready in:

Ingredients

- 450g lean rump steak
- 2 tbsp dairy and wheat-free Worcestershire sauce
- 2 tsp coarsely ground black pepper
- For the salad
- 250g 'Free From' fusilli pasta (we used Sainsbury's)
- 1 bunch spring onion, thinly sliced
- 3 red peppers, grilled to remove the skins, deseeded and thickly sliced
- small bunch basil, torn
- For the dressing
- 4 tbsp extra-virgin olive oil
- 2 tbsp sherry vinegar
- 2-3 tbsp freshly grated horseradish, to taste

Direction

- Marinate the steak in the Worcester sauce for 10 mins and sprinkle over the black pepper.
- Cook the pasta according to pack instructions, drain, then toss with the spring onions, peppers and basil. Mix the dressing ingredients together, season, then set aside.
- Heat the barbecue or a griddle pan until very hot. Cook the steak for 3 mins on each side, or until cooked to your liking. Cut into thick slices, then toss into the pasta with the dressing. Adjust seasoning to taste and serve.

Nutrition Information

- Calories: 498 calories
- Saturated Fat: 4 grams saturated fat
- Sugar: 10 grams sugar
- Total Fat: 18 grams fat
- Total Carbohydrate: 58 grams carbohydrates
- Fiber: 6 grams fiber
- Protein: 31 grams protein
- Sodium: 0.56 milligram of sodium

171.   Merlot Poached Pears With Vanilla & Cinnamon

Serving: 4 | Prep: 10mins | Cook: 1hours | Ready in:

Ingredients

- 750ml bottle Merlot or other red wine
- 200g golden caster sugar
- 2 cinnamon sticks, snapped in half

- 1 vanilla pod, halved lengthways then halved across to make 4 strips
- 4 firm pears, peeled

Direction

- Tip the wine, sugar, cinnamon and vanilla into a deep medium pan and heat gently until the sugar dissolves. Add the pears, making sure they are fully covered by the wine, then simmer for 30 mins until they are just tender. If the pears are very ripe, they may be ready in 20 mins. Can be made up to 2 days ahead – leave the pears in the syrup in the fridge until you're ready to finish the recipe.
- Remove the pears from the pan with a slotted spoon and boil the syrup for 30 mins to reduce it and make it more syrupy. Cool, then chill for up to 2 days. Remove from the fridge 1 hr before serving.

Nutrition Information

- Calories: 399 calories
- Sodium: 0.1 milligram of sodium
- Total Carbohydrate: 65 grams carbohydrates
- Sugar: 65 grams sugar
- Fiber: 4 grams fiber
- Protein: 1 grams protein

172. Miso Roasted Aubergine Steaks With Sweet Potato

Serving: 2 | Prep: 20mins | Cook: 1hours5mins | Ready in:

Ingredients

- 1 large aubergine (about 375g)
- 2 tbsp brown miso paste (we used Clearspring)
- 350g sweet potatoes, unpeeled and cut into chunky wedges
- 1 tbsp sunflower oil

- thumb-sized piece ginger, grated
- 1 garlic clove, grated
- pinch of pink Himalayan salt
- 8 spring onions, sliced diagonally
- small pack parsley, leaves chopped

Direction

- Heat oven to 180C/160C fan/gas 4. Peel the aubergine with a potato peeler and roughly spread the miso paste all over it – the best way to do this is with the back of a spoon.
- Put it in a roasting tin along with the sweet potato wedges. Pour 225ml boiling water into the base of the tin, then add the oil, ginger and garlic. Sprinkle a pinch of salt over the wedges and place in the oven.
- After 30 mins, pour another 125ml boiling water into the base of the tin and roast for another 20 mins. Repeat, adding 50ml boiling water and the spring onions, and roast for 10 mins more. Check the aubergine is cooked by inserting a knife in the centre – if it is ready it will easily slide in and out, and the aubergine will be soft on the inside.
- Sprinkle the chopped parsley over the potato wedges, slice the aubergine into 2cm thick 'steaks' and serve on top of the potatoes. If there is no sauce in the bottom of the tin, add 3 tbsp water to loosen up the miso, then pour the miso gravy over the aubergine steaks and sprinkle with cracked black pepper.

Nutrition Information

- Calories: 344 calories
- Total Fat: 8 grams fat
- Protein: 6 grams protein
- Sodium: 2.5 milligram of sodium
- Sugar: 30 grams sugar
- Total Carbohydrate: 54 grams carbohydrates
- Saturated Fat: 1 grams saturated fat
- Fiber: 15 grams fiber

173. Seafood Paella

Serving: 8 | Prep: 40mins | Cook: 1hours10mins |Ready in:

Ingredients

- 20-24 raw shell-on king prawns
- 2 tbsp olive oil
- 500g monkfish, cut into chunks
- 1 large onion, finely chopped
- 500g paella rice
- 4 garlic cloves, sliced
- 2 tsp smoked paprika
- 1 tsp cayenne pepper (optional)
- pinch of saffron
- ½ x 400g can chopped tomatoes (save the rest for the stock, below)
- 500g mussels, cleaned
- 100g frozen peas
- 100g frozen baby broad beans
- handful parsley leaves, roughly chopped
- For the stock
- 1 tbsp olive oil
- 1 onion, roughly chopped
- ½ x 400g can chopped tomatoes
- 6 garlic cloves, roughly chopped
- 1 chicken stock cube
- 1 star anise

Direction

- Peel and de-vein the prawns, reserving the heads and shells. Return the prawns to the fridge.
- To make the stock, heat the oil in a large pan over a medium-high heat and add the onion, tomatoes, garlic, and reserved prawn shells and heads. Cook for 3-4 mins, then pour in 2 litres of water and add the stock cube and star anise. Bring to a boil, then simmer for 30 mins. Leave to cool slightly, then whizz in batches in a blender or food processor. Strain through a fine sieve.
- Heat the oil in a large paella pan or an extra-large frying pan. Brown the monkfish for a few mins each side, then remove and set aside.

Add the onion and fry for 4-5 mins until softened.

- Stir in the rice and cook for 30 secs to toast. Add the garlic, paprika, cayenne (if using) and saffron, cook for another 30 secs, then stir in the tomatoes and 1.5 litres of the fish stock. Bring to the boil, then turn down to a simmer and cook, stirring, for about 10 mins (the rice should still be al dente). Return the monkfish to the pan with the prawns, mussels, peas and broad beans.
- Cover the pan with a large baking tray, or foil, and cook on a low heat for another 10-15 mins until the mussels are open and the prawns are cooked through. Scatter over the parsley before serving.

Nutrition Information

- Calories: 384 calories
- Fiber: 5 grams fiber
- Saturated Fat: 1 grams saturated fat
- Protein: 26 grams protein
- Total Fat: 6 grams fat
- Sugar: 5 grams sugar
- Total Carbohydrate: 54 grams carbohydrates
- Sodium: 1.5 milligram of sodium

174. Spiced Sweet Potato Wedges

Serving: 8 | Prep: 10mins | Cook: 40mins |Ready in:

Ingredients

- 2 tsp ground cumin
- 2 tsp chilli flakes
- 2 tsp sumac
- 2 tbsp thyme leaves, roughly chopped
- 2 tbsp rosemary leaves, roughly chopped
- 3 garlic cloves
- zest and juice 1 lemon
- 3 tbsp olive oil
- 1 ¼kg sweet potatoes, cut into wedges

Direction

- Heat oven to 200C/180C fan/gas 6. Using a pestle and mortar, bash together the spices, herbs, garlic and some seasoning.
- Spoon into a large bowl and stir in the lemon zest and juice, and the oil. Add the potatoes and toss together. Arrange, skin-side down, on 2 baking trays and bake for 30–40 mins until soft inside and crisp on the outside.

Nutrition Information

- Calories: 193 calories
- Sugar: 9 grams sugar
- Saturated Fat: 1 grams saturated fat
- Fiber: 5 grams fiber
- Sodium: 0.2 milligram of sodium
- Total Carbohydrate: 32 grams carbohydrates
- Protein: 2 grams protein
- Total Fat: 5 grams fat

175.   Vegan Crepes

Serving: Makes 6 small pancakes | Prep: 5mins | Cook: 25mins | Ready in:

Ingredients

- 125g gluten-free plain flour (we used Doves Farm)
- egg replacer, equivalent to 1 whole egg (we used Orgran No Egg) mixed with 2 tbsp water
- 250ml hemp or coconut milk (we tried Good Hemp and Koko)
- sunflower or rice bran oil, for frying
- orange segments and agave syrup, to serve

Direction

- Put the flour in a bowl and make a well in the centre. Pour in the Orgran egg replacer and a quarter of the milk.
- Use an electric whisk to thoroughly combine the mixture, then beat in another quarter of the milk. Once lump free, mix in the remaining milk. Leave to rest for 20 mins. Stir again before using.
- Heat a small non-stick frying pan with a splash of oil. When hot pour a small amount of the mixture into the pan and swirl around to coat the base – you want a thin layer.
- Cook for a few mins until golden brown on the bottom, then turn over and cook until golden on the other side. Repeat until you have used all the mixture, stirring the mixture between pancakes and adding more oil to the frying pan as necessary.
- Serve with an orange wedge and a drizzle of agave syrup or filling of your choice. This mixture keeps for a few days if you store it covered in the fridge. Give it a good whisk before using.

Nutrition Information

- Calories: 108 calories
- Fiber: 0.2 grams fiber
- Protein: 3.6 grams protein
- Total Fat: 3 grams fat
- Saturated Fat: 0.3 grams saturated fat
- Total Carbohydrate: 16.2 grams carbohydrates
- Sugar: 0.7 grams sugar

Index

A

Almond 4,65

Anise 4,75

Apple 3,4,5,19,30,37,47,48,56,82

Apricot 4,72,74

Asparagus 3,6,31

Aubergine 5,98

Avocado 3,27,30

B

Bacon 3,5,14,83

Banana 3,4,5,12,67,74,91,93,94

Barley 3,28

Basil 4,70

Beans 3,4,8,38,47

Beef 5,81,97

Beetroot 4,48,58

Berry 4,74

Blueberry 4,59

Brazil nut 58,91

Bread 5,91

Broccoli 3,10,23,38

Butter 3,4,5,12,49,67,82,87,94

C

Cake 4,5,58,59,60,61,62,63,64,66,68,69,88

Capers 3,23

Caramel 4,76

Carrot 3,4,26,60,64

Cauliflower 3,26,29

Celeriac 3,39

Celery 3,18

Cheese 4,79

Cherry 4,5,60,65,83

Chicken 3,4,5,27,31,32,36,39,41,52,83,84,86,87,89

Chickpea 3,4,26,40,45

Chicory 3,37

Chilli 3,31,32

Chips 3,11

Chocolate 4,5,61,62,66,71,93

Chorizo 5,82

Cider 3,39

Cinnamon 5,97

Coconut 3,4,5,8,17,33,59,83,93,94

Couscous 3,19

Cranberry 4,72

Cream 3,4,5,32,72,93

Crisps 4,47,56,57

Curry 3,4,5,33,34,35,40,45,46,54,83

Custard 4,68

D

Dijon mustard 28,81,93

Duck 4,51

E

Edam 4,43

Egg 3,5,6,7,9,10,11,14,18,82,100

English muffin 33

F

Fat 6,7,8,9,10,11,12,13,14,15,16,17,18,19,20,21,22,23,24,25,26,27,28,29,30,31,32,33,34,35,36,37,38,39,40,41,42,43,44,45,46,47,48,49,50,51,52,53,54,55,56,57,58,59,60,61,62,63,64,65,66,67,68,69,70,71,72,73,74,75,77,78,79,80,81,82,83,84,85,86,87,88,89,90,91,92,93,94,95,96,97,98,99,100

Fennel 3,17,23

Fish 3,5,33,34,85,88

Conclusion

Thank you again for downloading this book!

I hope you enjoyed reading about my book!

If you enjoyed this book, please take the time to share your thoughts and post a review on Amazon. It'd be greatly appreciated!

Write me an honest review about the book – I truly value your opinion and thoughts and I will incorporate them into my next book, which is already underway.

Thank you!

If you have any questions, **feel free to contact at:** *author@thymerecipes.com*

Caroline Riffe

thymerecipes.com

Printed in Great Britain
by Amazon